Professional Ethics and Primary Care Medicine

Professional Ethics
and Primary Care Medicine

Beyond Dilemmas and Decorum

Harmon Smith

Harmon L. Smith and Larry R. Churchill

Duke University Press   *Durham* 1986

For Olen R. Churchill, Mary C. Churchill,
and Harmon L. Smith III

Acknowledgments

This book issues from a collaboration between us which now extends over several years. Each of us, in his own university, has taught courses, offered seminars, conducted grand rounds, and otherwise consulted in the area of ethics and medicine. Occasionally we have been able to work together in undergraduate and postgraduate conferences for physicians and nurses, and sometimes in community-wide symposia. Much of that work focused, as most of the literature to date in this area has done, on high-technology tertiary care interventions.

Out of these experiences and their attendant reflections, and the frustration and prospect they engendered, we began to appreciate the possibilities for addressing these matters of such mutual and general interest in ways that could offer larger coherence and comprehensiveness than the currently governing approaches. The result is this book, for which we both lay full claim, which invites its readers to consider seriously a more generous—indeed, we think, a more appropriate—way to address these matters.

As with any undertaking of this sort, many persons have generously helped and we are glad now to be able to acknowledge their support. Albert Nelius, Mary Canada, and John L. Sharpe III, of the Perkins Library staff, together with Donn Michael Farris and Harriett V. Leonard, of the Duke University Divinity School Library, provided unfailing assistance with our bibliographic needs. Gail Chappell and Jean Oliver converted untidy drafts into intelligible typescript. Pamela L. Porter provided us excellent research assistance, and James F. Kirkley very helpfully composed the index.

We owe a special debt to our students—undergraduate, medical, divinity, doctoral, and postgraduate—who not only listened sympathetically and critically to our attempts to formulate the content of this book, but also taught us in important ways that only they may recognize. We are happy also to acknowledge the support and suggestions of several physician colleagues and co-teachers over the long time that this manuscript was aborning, particularly E. Harvey Estes, Daniel T. Gianturco, and Robert J. Sullivan of Duke, and James A. Bryan, Alan W. Cross, John J. Frey and C. Glenn Pickard of the University of North Carolina. Albert Keller and Alex Sanchez helpfully contributed two of the case studies.

Beyond these more particular debts, we gratefully acknowledge the less tangible but equally important contributions to our thinking by colleagues in the Departments of Social and Administrative Medicine and Religious Studies of the University of North Carolina at Chapel Hill and the Divinity School and Department of Community and Family Medicine of Duke University.

To Joanne Ferguson, Editor-in-Chief of the Duke University Press, whose enthusiasm for our work and patience in steering it through the editorial rapids never flagged, we are bound to say our special thanks.

We want, finally, to acknowledge the love and long-suffering of our families, whose affectionate understanding and support forwarded our work in ways that only recipients of such generosity can know and gladly affirm.

Contents

Introduction

A 46-year-old executive has been Dr. M.'s patient for several years. He is a chain smoker, and, despite frequent attempts at helping him to quit, he continues to smoke two packs a day. Finally, Dr. M. elects to send him a letter after a recent physical examination in which he states, "Upon reviewing your chest x-ray with a radiologist, there appears to be early evidence of emphysema." The chest x-ray is actually within normal limits.

The patient stops smoking cold and in subsequent follow-up visits remains indebted to Dr. M. for "changing his life."

For many the term "medical ethics" evokes an image of exotic life-or-death choices concerning abortion, euthanasia, care of malformed infants, human experimentation, and the like. To deal with such dilemmas, ethical principles are deployed, alternatives are listed, and choices are deduced that are thought to be consistent with the overriding principles.

This image betrays a superficial understanding of both ethics and medicine, and especially as these are the concern of the primary care physician. The popular understanding of medical ethics would have us ask of the above case: Was the physician right or wrong to deceive his patient? and, What principle(s) justify his action?

This case, however, does not depict a moral problem. It describes, instead, a relationship between a physician and a patient; and before we can hope to assess the physician's decisions and actions on moral grounds, we must ask some prior questions. How does each party perceive that relationship? How does the physician understand himself as a healer? What is his role? His obligation? On what (or whose) authority does he act? Likewise, what does the patient intend by his ongoing partnership with this doctor? What does he need? want? ask for? What perceptions of health/disease, independence/dependence, care/cure—among others—animate this relationship and make it (in whatever sense) a therapeutic alliance?[1]

Philosophers, lawyers, physicians, social scientists, and others have only recently addressed themselves to the broad range of issues which arise from medical care; and Protestant religious ethicists were only a few years earlier in their inquiries into these matters. On the other hand, Roman Catholic moral theology has long been attentive to medico-moral problems, and Judaism possesses a lengthy tradition of Rabbinic responsa and the dicta of religious courts on these subjects. The tendency of Jewish medical ethics, owing to classical methodology, has been to be case-oriented; and while Roman Catholic moralists have utilized carefully wrought principles for guidance, their tendency has been to be casuistic as well. Both of these approaches have come to be regarded as "legalistic," and, in much current discussion, rejected or disregarded.

Affirmations of secularity, in the sense that distinctly religious predicates are abandoned in favor of nonreligious reasoning, have doubtless influenced this shift. But beyond that has been the recognition that "legalist" systems—which seek to provide codes or lists of concrete rules for the direction of human behavior—are deficient for several reasons: (1) they too easily deteriorate into legalisms in which codes or rules are taken to be more important than persons; (2) no list of rules can ever be supposed to be complete enough or sufficiently sensitive to the vast and varied array of concrete situations; and, (3) legalist systems short-circuit the ethical task by asking only which rule applies in a given situation, thereby depriving actors of entering personally and creatively the situations within which they are expected to respond.

"Formal" systems contrast with code moralities in that they avoid building lists of answers to specific questions and attempt instead to provide general principles from which moral agents might design particular actions arising out of specific situations. This methodology has been prominent among contemporary philosophical and Protestant Christian treatments of issues in ethics and medicine—in the former case owing to recent interest in existentialism and linguistic analysis, and in the latter case deriving from the Reformation heritage which poses serious difficulty for treating religious obligation systematically in secular arenas.

As a result, purely formal systems are also problematic in several aspects: (1) their emphasis on individual autonomy in decision making fails to recognize important communitarian dimensions in customary human affairs; (2) they give insufficient support and direction to moral agents when they are confronted by bewildering complexity in almost every concrete choice; and (3) they tend to lapse into antinomianism—literally, lawlessness—inasmuch as in dispensing with codes there is a tendency also to dispense with firm principles.

By couching our questions, and the chapters which follow, as we do, we wish to affirm the person-centered character of medical ethics; that principles and rules reflect our assumptions about what relationships (and the people who form them) should be like. Hence, to jump from problems to principles or rules, and then to solutions, does violence to the very stuff that makes moral problems what they are. Medical-ethical problem-solving is not a generalizable and repeatable exercise in logic; it is an examination of the moral motivations and sensibilities which constitute us as "doctor" or "patient." Put another way, medical ethics is first and foremost about persons— what they intend, desire, and will, and especially what they value. The explicit acts of deciding and choosing are an important part, but only a part of ethics, and to focus on these exclusively is to distort ethics and reduce a complex moral life to only one of its aspects.

A standard critique of professional ethics in medicine has been that it is chiefly concerned with decorum and never rises above the level of etiquette to genuine ethical reflection. The work in medical ethics over the past decade has somewhat remedied this shortcoming by focusing upon moral dilemmas and emphasizing logic, rationality, and the application of general ethical principles to such cases. The results have given a new rigor to ethical analysis in medicine; but because the focus has been almost exclusively on problem solving, other facets of the moral life in medicine have been neglected and have fallen into disrepute.

Moral conflict at the decisional edge is now perceived to be the crux of medical ethics and is thereby thought to exhaust contemporary notions of morality. For example, a teacher of medical ethics can choose among such texts as *Contemporary Issues in Bioethics, Ethical Issues in Modern Medicine, Ethical Decisions in Medicine,* and *Case Studies in Medical Ethics,* to list only a few. The titles accurately convey the assumption of this mode of approach; moral aspects of biomedicine are to be couched as problems, stated in cases, which then issue into options suitable for a decision, which is finally justified by recourse to rules and/or principles.

We have mostly praise for these works, and we do not repeat in this essay the methods and strategies of problem solving which they successfully present. The difficulty with these and many similar works lies in their scope, and in the aspects of moral life which are neglected by their mode of approach. Ethics is more than rational processes and explicit decisions; it is also concerned with ideals, character, virtues, and various senses of self and the human situation.

Beauchamp and Childress,[2] who have written one of the best recent works in medical ethics, seem cognizant of the limitation of this approach. Their final two chapters are addressed to "Professional/ Patient Relationships" and to "Ideals, Virtues and Conscientious Actions." Yet even here it is too little, too late. The chapter on relationships is a discussion of the application of various moral rules, while ideals and virtues are treated as an afterthought. Nowhere is there real probing of moral sensibilities in mundane practice, before or after the big decisions, nor an acknowledgment that professional life has distinctive moral patterns which go beyond rules and principles.

The conventional stress on principles and rational decision procedures is ethics-at-a-distance. It eschews and avoids the complexity of medical self-perceptions, professional loyalties, and the subtle influences of habits of practice; so it ignores important dimensions of relationships. We believe that these unattended or omitted aspects lie at the very core of medical ethics, and that they affect profoundly the use of principles and the range of options which may be considered. In short, we are less concerned with the clarity of a physician's logic than with the figures of his moral imagination and his professional sense of self.

Instead of focusing upon modes of reasoning and criteria for moral judgments when a serious decision is at hand, we want to describe and assess the customs, traditions, and self-images of physicians. By this effort, we hope to invite students to reflect on their expectations and assumptions, and practitioners to reflect on their clinical experiences. This book is an invitation to do ethics in a more generous philosophical and humane (and medical!) sense than is possible in the conventional problem-solving approach.

All of this is intended to displace from the center of consideration the question: What should I do? To be sure, this question cannot be ignored; but it must be suspended temporarily in order for broader ethical reflection to occur.

It is especially in primary care that we see the inadequacy of treating professional ethics as merely rational problem-solving, on the one hand, or as expressions of etiquette and decorum, on the other. Primary care calls for an expanded medical ethics, with an enlarged process for dealing with specific problems and decisions, and a fuller sense of the professional norms which underwrite medicine's activities and give them social sanction.

Chapter 1, "Primary Care: A Moral Notion," provides foundational definitions of ethics and primary care which are developed more fully in subsequent chapters.

Chapter 2, "Ethics and Professionalism," traces the domination of science and the forces of professionalization over ethical thinking. We argue that ethical thinking in medicine has been largely usurped by these forces, and warped by the demands of a modern scientific ethos on questions of value. Professional ethics, we believe, conceived on these terms, is truncated and narrow.

In chapter 3, "Moral Imagination and Medicine," we present a revised concept of professional ethics. Here we argue that the goals of primary care bespeak the need for a post-Aesculapian professional ethics, that is, the need for a moral imagination which is informed more fully by patient experiences and social priorities for medical services. Consent is examined as a major index for this revised professional ethics.

Our purpose in chapter 4, "Case Studies in Primary Care," is to indicate how choosing and acting on choices are expressions of the larger moral sense of self in medicine. Our aim here is not to solve these problems, but to show how professional norms and values, together with patient sensibilities and social priorities, inform problem solving. We argue for ways of perceiving and thinking, not for specific answers.

Chapter 5, "Primary Care and Social Justice," is concerned with the inadequacy of current medical ethical norms to address the problems of distribution and availability of medical resources and services. We argue that emphasis on primary care provides a way of speaking to medicine's goals and purposes at this communal, macro-level, as well as at the individual, micro-level.

Our thesis throughout this essay is that "primary care" is not descriptive merely of the context of care, but of a different philosophy of medical care which embraces a normative purpose somewhat at variance with current customs and practices.

1 ◇ Primary Care: A Moral Notion

What Is Ethics?

In its broadest sense, *ethics* concerns how we live and what choices we make. As a particular professional expression of the larger discipline, *medical ethics* has to do with how physicians choose values and embody them in professional relationships with patients, families, colleagues, and the general public. On these terms, ethics is not unique to any person or group of persons but represents our common striving to make sense of those things we think and believe to be worthwhile, things which in turn we undertake to express in our actions and behavior.

Each of us is confronted, in the course of a normal day's activities, with a series of questions about what we ought to do, what would be the good or preferable choice, what is right or appropriate in this situation. The sum of the answers which a person (or group of persons) gives to these kinds of questions constitutes a system of *morals,* that is, a set of customary behaviors which are generally characteristic of that person (or group). The moral question always asks *what* to do.

But that exercise alone does not exhaust our interest in defining good or right or appropriate, because asking "what should I do?" logically entails answering another question: where do I turn to find out what is right and good and appropriate? This is properly an *ethical* query because it probes behind the "what" to the "why" in an effort to give defensible reasons for this choice or decision.

This process, which is very often taken for granted, is no less critical because it is so very familiar to us. For the most part, we tend to have enough shared assumptions about our values and their expression in actions that we do not need to articulate the process explicitly.

A physician, for example, may prescribe a certain drug for a certain diagnosis without going on to say what is clearly implied, namely, that he thinks your problem is X and he wants you to take Y because taking Y will correct X and result in Z.

Underlying the implied or tacit dimension of this relationship between physician and patient are several ingredients so essential that without them there would be no reason for these two to engage together in this transaction. These are all of those ways that both patient and physician suppose and expect that the answer given to "what should I do?" will be rooted in the anterior commitment of both to the patient's health and well-being. That is the presumptive operant value of Western medicine; that is the ethical dimension of the physician-patient relationship. Whatever the physician as physician may then "do" for or to or with the patient is thus referenced to this consensual and fiduciary bond, which authorizes a physician-patient relationship by accounting for "why" each ventures to do anything in concert with the other.

The consent of the general public to this "private" relationship is similarly authorizing; we approve, as it were, *what* is going on here because we sanction *why* it is going on here. Indeed, we can be relatively comfortable sometimes not knowing the "what" because the "why" is itself so trustworthy and secure. On the other hand, when we are given (or suppose that we have) reason to question "what" physicians are doing, our queries invariably and above all want to get at "why?" That is the preeminent question about the Nazi medical experiments, that is the bedrock question in every instance where medicine is suspected of "doing things it is unauthorized to do," that is the question which underlies the distinction between "clinical investigator" and "physician"—*what* is going on here is (at least tacitly, but usually explicitly) a function of *why* it should be permitted or prohibited. The ethical question always asks why, and it is a question which operates at a variety of levels: between a society and a profession, between a profession and its professionals, between a professional and a client.

Our simple illustration of diagnosis and prescription is not the only one, however, and sometimes the "what" question is so complex and subtle and novel that we are obliged to exhibit both it and the reasons "why" in quite explicit ways; ways that have become familiar to us in the wake of innovative high-technology interventions about which there are many questions from many quarters. While our conventional covenants may be able to cope fairly well with prescribing penicillin for pneumococcal pneumonia, cardiac homografts may engender a quarrelsome debate on many fronts, not the least of which will have to do with "why" this surgery is appropriate to do, whether it ought to be done, and the like.

Getting straight about what-do-you-do-and-why is important not only because it constitutes the basis for intentional relationships; it also matters to us to know ourselves; we believe Socrates' dictum that the unexamined life is not worth living. Were one to adopt a neo-Machiavellian morality, in which one exploits rather than serves the other, this would be a nonsensical way to talk. But the enduring traditions of Western civilization and Western medicine are rooted in such relational categories as trust and fidelity and compassion and caring; and that kind of language obliges us to look carefully at the ways in which our beliefs correspond with our behavior, at how our conduct is congruent with our character, at whether our actions embody our affirmed and articulated values.

At the outset we defined ethics, in its broadest sense, as having to do with how we live and what choices we make. Now we may say that ethics, more narrowly defined, is systematic examination of those values which inform and are embodied in our moral choices. The principal action of ethics is cerebral, and we seek to identify those values which we believe to be worthwhile and to understand why we cherish them. But ethics and morals are coimplicative of each other, as we have seen, and there are clear behavioral spinoffs from this cerebral activity inasmuch as part of the aim of ethics is to assist us to discriminate among competing choices and make the best one possible.

So even as we emphasize, for the sake of clarity and precision, that ethics extends beyond specific choices to acknowledgment of where we stand and what we affirm as worthwhile, we cannot forget that the concrete, practical embodiment and expression of these values is what allows us believably to say that we affirm them. That kind of reality testing, at least in our cultural heritage, already commits us to truth telling, candor, and honesty; conversely, that kind of analysis of facts for values predisposes us against hypocrisy (from the Greek, *hypokrisis:* seeming or appearing to be, pretending a role).

Ethics thus helps us to answer clearly whether there is correspondence and congruence and complementarity between what we believe and how we behave. It does this, in part, through both forward and backward movements which illuminate the choices we face and the history and circumstance out of which those choices emerge. The forward movement of ethics seeks clarity, definition, appropriate values and priorities, suitable ways and means, and good results which are wanted or intended by this (rather than some other) choice; its backward movement considers whether moral choices confirm or repudiate personal, social, and professional history, whether what's going on here is arguably discontinuous with this culture's most deeply held values or actually mediating the application (in whatever novel ways) of ancient values to modern moral dilemmas. The historical dimension holds special interest for ethics because values do not have their genesis or extension in an existential vacuum.

These, then, are some of the reasons for taking ethics seriously and part of the rationale for what we hope to achieve in this investigation into the ethics of primary care. As rational inquiry, ethical reflection will protect us from a kind of knee-jerk morality, a largely reflexive and selfish reaction to something or somebody else's initiating action. It will equip us both to initiate and to respond because ethics obliges us to consider our moral reflexes in view of a constellation of values and possible actions.

At a very practical level, ethical deliberation is a way of dealing rationally with disputes between persons without resorting to recrimination or violence. Moral discussions can preserve civility between disputing parties, and can even nourish a sense of community when moral discourse occurs appropriately.

Ethical reflection can be, moreover, an aid in the face of moral tragedy: sometimes we are confronted with choices we would prefer not to have to make, sometimes we realize that we would have acted differently if more care had been (or could have been) given to the choice we made. Advance awareness of tragic conditions, and the acknowledgment moreover that many of the choices in medicine are irreversible, invest ethical deliberations with a special importance and seriousness.

What Is a Moral Problem?

A recent study of medical education concluded that recourse to "the moral perspective" is typically made only as a last resort, only after the clinical and legal aspects of medical problems have been exhausted.[1]

Perhaps this is the result of the customs of tertiary-care training centers, where educational activities share time with research priorities and patient care. But the fact of the matter, as primary care vividly illustrates, is that both clinical and legal aspects are part of the "moral perspective"; and it is a mistake, despite the integrity which each of these aspects rightly claims for itself, to suppose that clinical, legal, and ethical aspects are autonomous or (worse!) mutually exclusive. Because this is a fairly typical practice, however, many ethical problems never reach the stage of formulation as ethical problems, and thereby remain invisible or get interpreted as technical or legal concerns.

Mr. and Mrs. C. were patients in Dr. K.'s family practice. In the course of annual physical examination, customary blood serology studies revealed that Mrs. C. was positive for gonorrhea. Mr. C.'s serology was negative. Dr. K. was troubled about how to manage this situation: Mrs. C. had not intended to reveal an extramarital affair to Dr. K., and would not have done so verbally; Mr. C. was also Dr. K.'s patient and should be protected from the infection; Dr. K. believed that he could not, however, violate the confidential relationship which was between himself and Mrs. C. by informing Mr. C. Dr. K. considered several alternatives, among which were drugs resistant to the gonococcus bacterium for Mr. C. and fabricating reasons why Mr. and Mrs. C. should abstain from sexual intercourse during the infectious period.

There are surely clinical aspects of this case that are essential for understanding what is going on here; and there may be legal aspects as well in terms of adultery and of conflict of interest and malfeasance of office if Mr. C. is not protected. But these constitute the basis for what is essentially a "moral perspective" in this case, and that is whether—and if so, in what sense—Mr. and Mrs. C. understand and intend themselves to be married to each other. Morally perceived, Mrs. C.'s infection is symptomatic of something in the relationship between these two gone wrong.[2]

Moral problems are not scientific or empirical problems. They cannot be solved by recourse to more sophisticated scientific methods, or by gathering more evidence. With the best scientific knowledge applied and all the available evidence in, moral problems are still problematic because they call for understanding and judgment based on values. That there are no effective remedies for many forms of cancer is a scientific and technical problem, but the management choices which ensue from this recognition of patient care limitation are frequently moral in nature.

Similarly, moral problems are not matters of aesthetics, manners, or taste. It may be objectionable to grovel in one's plate rather than use a fork, but it is not a moral fault to do so. Conversely, it may be pleasing to use shiny and sterile instruments in an operating theater, and it is a moral fault not to do so. Moral questions carry a deep sense of obligation and oughtness; at their heart they evoke a sense that goodness is at stake.

But moral problems are frequently in jeopardy of being transmitted into other forms which trifle with goodness. Most often in our experience with physicians this occurs through "eliding," or slurring over, morally significant data and recasting it in another mold. There is a morally significant difference, for example, between observing that "she's keeping Lent" and "she's dieting," and that difference is simply the difference between fasting for religious purposes and dieting *qua se.* The action may, in each instance, appear to be the same; but, of course, it cannot be because different consequences are intended. It is no more the object of a religious fast to lose weight than it is the purpose of a diet to increase communion with God, and the consequences of these actions are skewed if their intentions are ignored.

So we should not confuse morally significant *concepts* and morally significant *acts.* Indeed, Eric D'Arcy insists that "certain kinds of acts are of such significance that the terms which denote them may not . . . be elided into terms which (a) denote their consequences, and (b) conceal, or even fail to reveal, the nature of the act itself."[3]

While it may be morally trivial to quibble over whether "he flicked the switch" or "he turned on the lights," it is a very different and morally serious matter if the switch he flicked carried out capital punishment by electrocution. Similarly, there is an important difference between saying "she has a genitourinary tract infection" and "she has gonorrhea."

In a recent discussion of managing the manner and time of human dying and death, one of the physicians present was greatly offended at the insensibility of those who would expedite the decision to allow-to-die by immediate stoppage of life-support systems. In our hospital, he said, we practice a "gradual turndown" of the machines.[4] This physician was uncomfortable with his role in these matters—so much so that he refused, even after having done all of the appropriate consultations and having been requested by nurses and advised by the hospital attorney, to write orders for a gradual turndown or "No CPR" or anything pertaining to this decision on the patient's chart— and thought that by the invention of a euphemism he could conceal the nature of the act itself.

It is not because there is such enormous evil or unfairness or even unkindness in eliding event into meaning that we condemn that way of talking; it is rather that the events are so significant for discriminating moral meaning that we need to preserve appropriate distinctions between them. Thus, Paul Ramsey points out that

Killing a man may or may not be murder, depending on the constitutive circumstances, i.e., those constituting murder. . . . Cutting off a man's leg may be mayhem or surgery. . . . There are, in short, specifying circumstances and non-specifying circumstances. Some circumstances may *constitute* the act, some may *change* the proper description of an act from one species to another . . . and some circumstances may cause an action to belong also to another moral species, as when a lie is also perjury, and finally there are some circumstances that are extenuating, aggravating, enhancing, or disentitling in the matter of attributing moral worth.[5]

The point is that *how* human actions are described is a part of moral discernment and, to a large measure, sets the stage for making moral decisions.

As value issues are reduced, by eliding or other means, to legal or technical or scientific judgments, the "sense of goodness" is eroded and eventually lost, eliminating the moral edge of a problem by disguising it and prohibiting its consideration as a moral problem. Radical feminists, for example, talk of abortion as though it were solely a political issue—in something of the same way that some gynecologists treat abortion as though it were altogether a medical matter. In each case, the moral significance of the act is reduced: on the one hand to a demand for unimpeded access to medical services, and on the other hand to a question of proper medical technique. To be sure, there are proper political and medical aspects to abortion; but neither of these modes of understanding, nor both of them together, exhaust the moral significance of the action or its consequences.

Positively defined, a moral problem is one in which values conflict; and that means that morally significant problems occur within a constellation of values. Resolutions to moral problems occur as persons make choices based on their assessment of values, that is, when they can make the constellation a commonwealth and choose a course of action because—at least for the persons deciding and choosing—it is the right one to embody these values. Whether the choice is technically correct or scientifically valid may well be part of the process by which many values in conflict and competition get sorted out, but neither of these ways of assessment constitutes the *conditio sine qua non* of moral judgment. Moral choices call on us to rank our values and espouse some or one of them over others. Physicians, for example, are traditionally thought to value both the relief of suffering and the preservation of life, but there are situations in which suffering can be relieved only at the eventual expense of life itself, or life preserved only at a cost of great personal distress and pain. Lawyers are supposed to have the highest respect for law and, simultaneously, to serve the ends of justice; but all of us, and perhaps especially legal positivists, know that while these may be simultaneous, they are hardly synonymous, professional duties. The love of God is free and unconditioned, clergy teach and preach; but the maintenance of institutionalized religion is not even cheap, much less free.

Moral problems are of this sort, where affirmation runs headlong into action which minimally calls for interpretation (and maximally threatens compromise of the integrity of the affirmation), where alternative behaviors threaten our cherished beliefs, where character is made vulnerable to conduct. The heart of a moral problem is that cluster of competing and conflicting values, all of which the moral agent wants to affirm but only some of which can be selected as bearing and embodying the agent's moral commitments in this circumstance. The existential philosophers and novelists of this century have insisted that we *are* our choices, that we become what we choose. We resist this too-simple equation; all the same, it is accurate to say that part of the sense of gravity which we associate with moral choices stems from our recognition that who we are is irrefragably communicated and reflected in our moral choices. So while Plato was correct to say that "being" is anterior to "doing," it would be a mistake not to acknowledge the ways in which "doing" both expresses and invariably shapes "being." Moral choices affirm or violate our sense of self as most kinds of choices do not, and that is why moral choices are critical choices: they appeal to the sort of person we are and aspire to become.

Ethics is frequently identified with moral problem-solving and, indeed, this is an important aspect of ethics. Ethics is crippled and incomplete without concrete and specific decisions and actions. Moreover, most of us think about ethics only when we are confronted with a moral perplexity. Many texts on ethics begin with a set of problems (and move quickly to principles) for precisely this reason. But sooner or later problems and principles must refer back to the structure of the moral imagination and to the larger sensibility in which decisional elements take shape.

Our focus in this volume is upon the moral imagination of physicians, that is, upon the character, sense of integrity, ideals, and virtues of practitioners. Ethical reflection at this level is not so much concerned with problems to be solved as with lives to be lived. It is this aspect of ethics which shows itself before and after decisions are made, in how the professional task is perceived, in the assumptions about which choices are possible, and in the routine ways that values nourish and inform professional life. Who are physicians? Who are patients? What relationships should obtain between them? What purposes should medicine serve? These are among the basic value questions we will probe. Specific ethical problem-solving will finally be grounded in how these larger questions are answered. We are especially concerned, therefore, with how recent concepts of primary care impinge upon these fundamental questions.

What Is Primary Care?

The self-definitions of professionals are, in irreducibly important ways, prominent in their perceptions of right and wrong, good and evil, appropriate and inappropriate. Increasingly these understandings of who one is and how one is expected to act—as a professional—are contained in codes of ethics (which are misnomers), or principles of ethics, or codes of professional responsibility which have been formulated and formally adopted by the professional organization. So there is The Code of Ethics for Engineers, the Principles of Medical Ethics of the American Medical Association, and the Code of Professional Responsibility of The American Bar Association. In each case, the purpose of the document is to make explicit, and binding upon affiliated members, the profession's concept of itself as moral agent.

There is not yet a formal statement of the ethics of primary care, but enough has been published to advance the claim that there is increasingly a broad, tacit consensus within medicine about what primary care is and what it ought to do. Here are some of the definitions. Albert and Charney held that primary care is not synonymous with comprehensive medicine, social medicine, preventive medicine, community medicine, personal medicine, ambulatory medicine, or family medicine; these terms overlap with primary care but cannot be used interchangeably with primary care. Primary care medicine is first-contact medicine which assumes longitudinal responsibility for the patient, regardless of the presence or absence of disease, and serves as the "integrationist" for the patient.[6]

Janeway described the fundamental scientific base of primary care as health promotion, identification of individuals at special risk, early detection of serious disease, management of acute emergencies, and the ability to render continuing care to chronicallly ill patients.[7]

In 1975, Silver and McAtee offered a descriptive definition of the scope and content of primary care: "Primary health care includes the initial contact of the patient with the health care system and is high-quality, comprehensive, individualized, quickly responsive, and readily accessible care that is patient-oriented, easy to use, and based on a firm foundation which integrates knowledge of the medical, biological, physical, social, psychological, and behavioral sciences."[8]

Petersdorf elaborated similar themes in defining the primary care physician as being in first contact, making initial assessment and attempting to solve as many of the patient's problems as possible, coordinating health care team consultants and ancillary personnel, remaining in contact with the patient as advisor and confidante, and assuming continued responsibility for care.[9]

Rather than define primary care in terms of the knowledge and skills of a particular kind of physician, or in terms of the severity or incurability of the patient's illness, or in terms of first-contact care, Millis defined primary care as including "all the health services needed by a given population that are *not* provided by secondary and tertiary care."[10]

Rogers, however, reiterated a description of primary care in terms of first contact and continuing responsibility for comprehensive care, ordinarily within a defined geographic area, and for groups of people who are usually ambulatory and able to function at home.[11]

In another essay, Rogers amplified these notions and emphasized that primary care entails longitudinal attention for groups (not just individuals) in terms of social and psychological factors which contribute to illness, along with concern for physiological and disease-oriented aspects. This kind of care is, of necessity, given by several kinds of physicians (internists, pediatricians, obstetricians, gynecologists, family practitioners) and other health professionals (nurses, physician assistants, HMOs, et al.).[12] Any primary care system, he continues, must have certain capabilities:

(1) It must provide ready access to the physician or some other health professional who can cope effectively with ordinary medical problems. (2) It must be able to separate from the many innocent-appearing situations those few that are potentially serious and it must provide properly for them. (3) It must provide scientific, humanistic support to those that it serves. (4) It must provide care on a continuing basis. (5) It must be distributed with reasonable equity. (6) As a system, it must be stable and self-renewing, i.e., those who work in it must enjoy it and others must wish to enter the field. (7) It must have a proper fit with the way of life or the culture of those it serves, and this will vary widely by background, culture, and locale in our diverse and far-flung country. (8) It must be able to receive support in competition with other real needs of our society.[13]

As early as 1974, under the auspices of the Ontario Ministry of Health, primary care was defined as including "not only those services that are provided at first contact between the patient and the health professional but also responsibility for promotion and maintenance of health and for complete and continuous care for the individual including referral when required."[14]

In 1976, the American Academy of Family Physicians offered its definition: "Primary care is a type of medical care delivery which emphasizes first contact care and assumes ongoing responsibility for the patient in both health maintenance and therapy of illness. It is personal care involving a unique interaction and communication between the patient and the physician. It is comprehensive in scope, and includes the overall coordination of the care of the patient's health problems, be they biological, behavioral or social. The appropriate use of consultants and community resources is an important part of effective primary care."[15]

An emerging consensus was clearly on the horizon in 1977 when the Committee on Standard Terminology of the North American Primary Care Research Group published "A Glossary for Primary

Care." Although the NAPCRG's definitions are not original but modifications of earlier statements by other groups, they do stand as a kind of benchmark: "Primary care is a type of health care which emphasizes first-contact care and assumes ongoing responsibility for the patient in both health maintenance and therapy of illness; it is personal care involving a unique interaction and communication and includes the overall coordination of care of the patient's health problems with the appropriate use of consultants and community resources."[16]

With the publication in 1978 of the Institute of Medicine's study report on "A Manpower Policy for Primary Health Care," the process by which primary care has achieved its modern self-understanding is probably complete. This report defines primary health care as "accessible, comprehensive, coordinated, and continual care provided by accountable providers of health services (as distinguished from public, environmental, and occupational health services), where initial professional attention is paid to current or potential health problems. Frequently, primary care is associated with care of the 'whole person' rather than care for an illness."[17]

Owing to differing roles, and differing kinds of responsibility that are fitting for different patients in different circumstances, it is important that primary care physicians and other health professionals have as clear as possible an understanding of who they are and what they are expected to do.

Primary care pediatricians and family doctors, for example, may have especially complicated relationships, and therefore privileges and responsibilities, to families as whole families, to minors, or to children who are too young to make their own voices heard in a decision. There are ordinarily additional factors, moreover, which further influence this dimension of moral judgments: the customs of the community, one's professional peers, legal considerations, and the seriousness of the consequences for the patient and/or the family. All of these together bespeak the pragmatic advantage of having some guidelines which assist in getting one's professional bearings. The analogy of the marine navigator may be apposite: one cannot plot a course until one's position is known. That is itself a value—in this case, directed purpose or purposive direction—which already signifies why a common self-understanding is desirable.

Although the IOM statement is not a code of ethics in any formal sense, it has moral implications which far exceed conventional formulations of moral agency in the practice of medicine.

Some Implications

All of the statements which we have briefly examined embody ethical positions; so while the IOM statement is fundamentally a moral assertion of the values which should inform primary care medicine, it is not unique in this respect. What is significantly different about the IOM statement is that the key term here is *not* "care of the 'whole person.' " That term has, of course, been much used; but while it is laudatory as a concept, it has also come too frequently to designate a loose cluster of ideologies. The key terms in the IOM statement are "accessible, comprehensive, coordinated, and continual care provided by accountable providers. . . ." To be sure, these phrases may also be seen as empty hortatory embellishments, not to be taken seriously, and in no way altering medicine's role in society. That will be most likely to occur if these phrases are filtered through current professional assumptions and self-definitions; in that event, they will go limp and lose any independent reference point in their own right. To put it plainly: if physicians alone decide what counts as "accessible, comprehensive, coordinated, and continual care," these terms will lose their essential reference points, namely, the concerns of patients and the larger public.

It deserves saying clearly and directly that a corresponding move by "consumer advocate" and "patient rights" supporters will have a similarly disabling effect. The answer to Aesculapian authority is not populism.

The temptation to do just that sort of tampering with professional and popular referencing will be strong; indeed there are many evidences of it already. Why this is so, and why we believe that such an approach will not suffice, is explored in the following chapter. If this temptation can be resisted, and if the discussion of these terms can take place in a larger social and communal context, conventional medical ethics will have to shift to accommodate the significance of patient and societal, as well as innovative medical, factors. It is toward this shift and its benefits that we argue in the remainder of this book.

In the previous chapter we have discussed ethics and primary care in a general way. We have seen that the definition of primary care is it-self moral in nature, outlining as it does a set of responsibilities and duties for physicians in the provision of care and evoking a new im-age for the physician. But this new image is not yet in accord with current views of professional ethics in medicine. Why this is so re-lates to modern Western perceptions of science, of ethics, and of pro-fessionalism. We argue in this chapter that modern ethical sensibili-ties have been largely subverted by a professional ethics which has effectively foreclosed any broad, extra-professional sense of "the good." Taking ethics and primary care seriously means that questions of "the good" must be reopened.

Modern Science, Human
Self-Perceptions, and Ethics

One of the common, and widely held, notions in Western culture is that what distinguishes us from other animals is intelligence—or if not intelligence as a quantum difference, then at least the capacity (so far as we can tell!) to display our intelligence in rationally ex-plicit ways. Indeed, we are alleged to be *homo sapiens*. But that may be a label which is less descriptive of us-as-we-are than ambitious for us-as-we-would-like-to-be. Many of us would nowadays prefer to be thought reasonable than wise, perhaps because reasonableness is broadly believed to be requisite to wisdom as well as because *ratio* is within our reach in ways that *sapientia* is not. Since the Renaissance, *homo ratio* is probably the phrase which more accurately describes us-as-we-are. It follows that why we do what we do is amenable to rational constructs which account for both our behavior and the reasons for it.

That this way of accounting for ourselves is generally regarded as comforting does not diminish the ways in which it is a seriously overdrawn and fundamentally mistaken account of ourselves. If we were that kind (and only that kind) of creature, we would be able always to appeal to a rational rule or principle as the plain and sufficient warrant for our choices. But we patently are not that kind (and only that kind) of creature. We are simultaneously much grander and much less exalted than that. We appeal to reason, to rules, to principles, to be sure; but in the final analysis, these are probably much less the determinants and shapers of our behavior than they are the explicit accounting we choose to give for it. All the same, we continue to appeal to *ratio,* or to put it another way, to display ourselves as professionals rather than as persons.

To comprehend how we have thus ventured to account for ourselves and our actions—who we are and why we do what we do— would involve a long and thorough examination of Western intellectual history since the sixteenth century. While a full account is beyond our limited purposes here, we can gain a useful understanding by brief reference to the history of scientific method in Western thought.

Prior to the sixteenth and seventeenth centuries scientific method was virtually equated with the method of mathematical abstract science, which was itself indistinguishable from the method of deduction and syllogism which Aristotle had developed. For Aristotle the truth began with valid postulates (which he thought were self-evident), from which valid conclusions were then logically inferred. So there was an initial element of intuition, the valid postulates, and science was the sum of valid judgments which derived from those postulates.

From his time (384–322 B.C.) until the sixteenth century, Aristotle dominated Western intellectual history; but in the sixteenth century, a new conception of science emerged. The first step was Galileo's application of mathematics to physical bodies (which Aristotle had said could not be done); and the second step was Francis Bacon's definition of the scientific method of inquiry.[1] Of these two (Galileo and Bacon) Bacon's contribution is more pertinent to our interests here.

Bacon defined the scientific method of inquiry as first observation and then experimentation or manipulation. Thus induction, and not the deductive method of Aristotle, became the accepted procedure. What counts, according to Bacon, is observation of phenomena and reduction of the many variables to what is essential. So Bacon saw things as not significantly explained if explained in terms of their *telos* or end. A teleological explanation may provide a rational construction of things. Yet it is quantitative measurement and finding out how things happen, together with the laws and causes for why they happen, that puts into man's hands the power to manipulate and control things to his own ends. So the criterion of significance for Bacon was utility: a thing is significant in the measure to which it can advance human dominion.

Moreover, since truth is now the truth of the empirical experimental method, nothing can qualify as knowledge which is not arrived at by the experimental method. Thus ethical theory, aesthetics, history, and the like are either seriously questioned or entirely ruled out of the court of credibility. The result over the past three hundred years, and especially since the enlightenment of the mid-eighteenth century, is that ethics and moral philosophy, together with humanistic disciplines generally, have been largely relegated to ambiguity, uncertainty, or dubiety. Accordingly, truth and knowledge belong exclusively to the empirical experimental method. This explains why every candidate for the presidency nowadays has his own pollster to identify the political issues for particular constituencies. That is also why Flip Wilson's celebrated phrase—"what you see is what you get"—is, far from being comic nonsense, the first article of the creed bequeathed to us by Francis Bacon.

The effect of Bacon, and more generally the impact of modern experimental modes of knowledge, upon human self-perceptions has been profound. Only knowledge which is empirically testable is acceptable. The result has been either to discredit ethics altogether as hopelessly subjective, or to reduce ethics to rational decision processes. In the former case, ethics is no better than groundless superstition, emotionalism, or sheer opinion—all those characterizations that are ordinarily designated as *relativism*. In the latter case, ethics is no more than rule-governed "behavior." If this latter tactic is employed, ethics is salvaged, but at a severe price. Rules are thought to appeal to reason, and "behavior" is thought to be publicly observable, hence quantifiable and measurable. Ethics is thereby thought to be "scientific," but it is also reduced to only a shadow of what we all commonly take to be the moral life. All one has here are rules and behavior, but without the larger context of perceptions of value, motives, and intentions of human choices. This view is usually designated, in a generic way, as moral *absolutism*. This particular form is a scientific absolutism which tries to make ethics a collection of observable and objective facts and procedures about human choices.

As we argued in the first chapter, these accounts of ethics, and of human self-perceptions, are profoundly mistaken. Our location of rules and principles within a larger constellation of elements in a decision process is calculated to diminish the impact of these accounts, and also to diminish the prominence of rules and principles. Rules and principles are, we believe, actually subsidiary to professional role definitions, loyalties, and perceptions. So we turn now to these matters, in order to take a more detailed look at the traditional role of the physician and later on to examine the appropriateness of this role for primary care. The assumptions which underlie this traditional role form a portion of the character of the physician, and they therefore prominently influence the shape of routine professional activities. In a word, they constitute the dimension of ethics which is sometimes referred to as "character ethics," that is, those tacit norms which pattern and mold action and habit especially when one is engaged in customary practice. Because it is these tacit norms which shape routine actions, they are all the more powerful authorities for the ethics of the physician. Why this is so will become clear as we examine our terms.

Professional Ethics

The major Western philosophical traditions have encouraged us to think of ethics almost entirely in terms of rules, or principles, or codes of rational conduct. In this framework, ethics is viewed as a study of the rational processes for deciding the best course of action in situations of values conflict. To arrive at such decisions, we are told that we must employ rules, principles, maxims, codes, or moral formulae. But one of the liabilities of this notion is to challenge the credibility of ethics by making it appear to be a wholly abstract, mental process. The fact of the matter, as we argued earlier, is that ethical reflection is always mediated through the practical situation in which values-in-conflict arise, and for which an ethical choice has concrete and specific application and consequence. That is why, for example, ethical questions arise in different ways for doctors and lawyers: there is a significant divergence in the *practical* contexts of their work.

Indeed, the very formulation of ethical questions is shaped by the context of one's work and the contours of one's community of co-workers (what we sometimes call an *ethos*). The word "ethics," as also "ethos," is derived from the Greek ἠθικός which referred to customary behavior. To speak of ethics, then, is to speak of those regular and constant traits of character which identify actors and their actions. Similarly, ἦθος (ethos) was an accustomed place; that is, in our context, the practical setting within which ethical questions arise and in terms of which morally significant decisions are taken. The language itself suggests a close association between the character of work in a community and the scope of the community's resources for ethical reflection.

"Profession" is the second key term in our analysis. Perhaps it is useful at the outset to be reminded that "profession" was historically a vow made upon entrance to a religious order. Indeed, it is still customary to speak of the time when novitiates will make their profession and thereby become fully initiated into the order. But in the late seventeenth century, when industry had become highly specialized and the artisans of a given trade or craft had formed themselves into guilds, "profession" became secularized. Whereas the word had formerly identified the "three classic professions" (law, medicine, and divinity), it now came to mean "to be duly qualified" for any vocation or occupation in which professed knowledge of some branch of learning is used in an application to the affairs of a clientele. So "profession" nowadays is variously defined so as to include virtually any occupation from athletics to zymurgy. All the same, there are some principal features, colloquial usage notwithstanding, which consistently appear in both sociological studies and "professional" literature.

One of those characteristics is the distinction between "providers" and "performers," which holds that while business *provides* goods *to* a customer and trade *provides* service *for* a purchaser, a profession *performs* service *on* a client. More pertinent to our interests are all those ways in which a profession is "self-defined," roots its work in cerebral activity, controls qualification and training requirements for practitioners, is self-regulating, and usually is cloaked in the mystique of language and apparel. The most frequently cited marks of a modern profession are (1) that it have a theoretical knowledge base, (2) that it be designed for a special service, (3) that it exercise control of the service through control of the precursory knowledge and skill (i.e., professional education) needed to dispense it, (4) that it control the application and use of its knowledge and skill through licensing and accreditation, and (5) that it control the dispensation of its service.

These internal characteristics of a profession derive originally from a social mandate to provide a particular service. The profession's authority is thus vested in it by society's respect for and deference toward the specialized knowledge, skill, and service which, in turn, society wants. In sum, this means that a profession's *mandate to be* lies in a *service* need perceived by *society,* but that the profession's *license to act* lies in a *knowledge and skill* base which *it alone controls.* Society therefore looks to a profession for special knowledge, special skills, special resources, and special responsibilities. In return the profession is granted special authorities and powers.

Because self-organization and self-regulation are essential aspects of a profession, it follows that accountability to professional peers is a critical element. Having received society's mandate, professions also accept the superordinate function of assessing and governing themselves, on the supposition that no one outside the profession has sufficient knowledge or experience (and hence authority) to do so. This self-imposed accountability to peers constitutes the basis for collegiality within the profession as it functions to set standards for "good" professional practice and the development of career lines within the profession.

An example from nursing education illustrates this point well. Entering nursing students are typically very highly motivated to "help," to provide a needed and useful "service" for patients. But one of the early, and usually painful, lessons which student nurses learn is that service is performed through assignments. With that shift in the meaning of service comes a new relationship to patients and a new self-understanding. Nurses do not serve patients "directly" but through accepted professional *forms* of service, and it is professional prerogative to specify these forms, and by so doing to define patient needs, what constitutes service, whether an assignment is beneficial, and so on.

Francis Bacon once said that every man is held a debtor to his profession, a dictum which gives explicit notice to the binding obligations of the individual to the organized professional body which judges that individual's skill and merit. The obligations of a professional to the profession approach an allegiance which is religious in its depth of commitment, if not in its content. So it is well also to note the absence, in Bacon's dictum, of any sense of indebtedness to the society which initially authorizes and needs the exercise of professional knowledge and skill. It would appear that service to one's profession is repayment of a legitimate debt, but that service to one's patients or the general public carries no such corresponding obligation. That is a notion in Western medicine which is at least as old as the Hippocratic Oath, and it is clearly expressed there in terms of intraprofessional fealty. It is also a notion which allows George Bernard Shaw's aphorism to be fitting commentary: every profession, he said, is a conspiracy against the laity.

Medicine is in many ways the paradigm for a modern profession. Physicians hold great power in the health care system, the strength of their professional organization is unequaled, and the esteem and authority they are granted by the public remains high. Even when physicians are criticized as a group, as individuals they usually retain the confidence of their patients. (It is, after all, other people's doctors who are sometimes alleged to be incompetent or careless—but not mine!)

The Professionalization of Ethics

These comments would be unnecessary and inappropriate if it were not the case that professional ethics has tended to become a *professionalization of ethics*. Or, to put it more fully, professionalization narrows the scope of moral discernment because it diminishes, by rendering ineffectual, the personal (i.e., nonprofessional) resources for ethical reflection. This narrowing tendency, we contend, is especially evident in medicine. Paul Ramsey has said that "there is no profession which comes close to medicine in its concern to inculcate, transmit and keep in constant repair its standards governing the conduct of its members."[2]

Additional witness to medicine's professional strength is provided by the physical, emotional, and intellectual commitment exacted from those who seek entrance into the profession. That medical students learn standards of conduct, redefine the parameters for moral choices, and experience a reorientation of their value systems is a truism. Louis Lasagna put it well when he said that in the pragmatic, frenetic existence of medical education the student "may quickly absorb the moral atmosphere around him without questioning it."[3] And Edmund Pellegrino adds to the characterization by describing this moral atmosphere as relying too often upon "apodictic statements and simplistic solutions."[4] Indeed, the sociological studies conducted by the Columbia group in the 1950s identified the social organization of medicine as a critical determinant of a medical student's self-concept and values.[5]

While the powerful forces of professionalization in medicine clearly engender a deep sense of morality—what is right/wrong, good/bad, appropriate/inappropriate—it is important to ask about the scope and fit of this moral sensibility. We need to ask in particular whether this moral sensibility includes the capacity to step outside the customs and traditions engendered in medical training to inquire into the goodness of the professional value commitments themselves. That is not a gratuitous query, if only because there are certain notions, prominent within both Western civilization and Western medicine, which qualify as "universal norms." One of these, for example, is sanctity of life; another is egalitarianism. The social and political organization of the United States is largely built upon these notions; and the Nuremberg Code, the Declaration of Helsinki, and numerous other documents in the history of medicine, commit—sometimes tacitly, but frequently quite explicitly—medical policy and practice to these norms for authentication and legitimation.

The foundational documents of the United States state clearly that "We hold these truths to be self-evident, that all men [and women!] are created equal, and endowed by their Creator with certain inalienable rights"; that "No person shall be . . . deprived of life, liberty, or property without due process of law"; nor shall any state "deny to any person within its jurisdiction the equal protection of the laws."[6]

Or, from the Hippocratic Oath: "I will give no deadly medicine to anyone if asked, nor suggest any such counsel. . . . Into whatever houses I enter, I will go into them for the benefit of the sick, and will abstain from every voluntary act of mischief and corruption." Or, from the Declaration of Geneva (adopted by the World Medical Association in 1948, and reaffirmed as the basis for the Declaration of Helsinki in 1964): "the health of my patient will be my first consideration. . . . I will not permit considerations of religion, nationality, race, party politics, or social standing to intervene between my duty and my patient; I will maintain the utmost respect for human life, from the time of conception; even under threat, I will not use my medical knowledge contrary to the laws of humanity."

This is but a fraction of the evidence which could be multiplied many times over; but even this much demonstrates that there are substantial warrants for arguing the status of sanctity of life and egalitarianism as "universal norms." We could add that we have yet to meet a physician or nurse who, if allowed to say what they interpret these norms to mean, would fail to affirm them. What is less agreed upon these days is the depth and scope of these norms for guiding professional practice.

Professions are currently not inclined to have as a part of their animating spirit an outlet to a broader sphere, a self-examining principle. It is more common for ethical reflection to be filtered through the mores of the profession. Indeed, it is not infrequently held that special norms, or a special process of balancing norms, exists for a professional group because expertise in ethical decision-making resides in the members of that profession by virtue of the skills, experiences, or sensitivities acquired by entry into that profession. That presumption, incidentally, also underlies the claim that disputes involving professional practice should be adjudicated entirely by the profession. Clearly these attitudes are not the sole possession of medical professionals; but they are prominent enough to warrant attention specifically directed to medical professionals.

Arthur Dyck has suggested that the current widespread interest in and concern for ethics and health care derives from two mutually reinforcing causes for alarm: on the one hand is medicine's departure from traditional values, and on the other hand is the stifling of technological promise by adherence to traditional values.[7] Perhaps it is only stating the obvious; all the same we think it worth noting that the adversaries in this matter are not simply physicians versus the lay public, or scientists versus humanists, or any other neat division of the house. The fact is that people line up on one or another side of this debate irrespective of professional identity and role.

As a matter of record, there appears to be an emerging consensus that many kinds of judgment and expertise are needed if professions are to retain their integrity as professions. Thus Robert Veatch has argued that it is logically and logistically impossible to defer every decision to the layman. This does not mean, however, that the decision reverts to the professional in his professional role because of his superior technical skills, his unique set of norms, or his superior ability in reaching ethical judgments. It may revert to him—it must in some cases—but it will revert to him as another human being with no necessarily superior decision-making skills. . . . A system of decision-making which is rooted in a universal, human ethic may still call on the professional to make many decisions; it certainly will insist that he practice his trade ethically; but the decisions he makes will be made within a universal frame of reference, one which is not unique to the profession he is practicing. The conclusion to which I am led is that medical ethics must not be thought of as a special "professional ethic" at all, but as a specific application of the universal norms of ethical action.[8]

Since medicine as a profession claims so much of a person's time and energy and resources, it is not surprising that the moral ethos of doctors should be quite strong in resisting what is perceived to be an alien influence. We are not claiming, of course, that physicians are unresponsive to an ethics of the common good more diverse than that of the professional good. Physicians have always had the well-being of their patients as a principle of their codes, from Hippocrates to the present. It is how that as yet empty term, "well-being," is to be filled that is crucial. The hallmark of professionals is that they reserve for themselves the formulation of this definition, not only in its explicit content but also with reference to the criteria by which a content may be determined. In short, our claim is that professionalism in medicine tends not only to define "the good," but also to specify at a deeper level how definitions of "the good" are to be reached.

The ethos of professionalism in medicine constitutes a powerful set of assumptions, and has shaped the ethics of physicians in significant ways. The result is what we term the professionalization of ethics. Ethics—far from remaining the broad process of thinking which was presented earlier—has tended to be a somewhat insular and domesticated process, dominated by an attenuated professional mentality and culture.

But to say only that the ethics of medical professionals has been too narrow is to miss the point. The narrowness, the constriction, has to do with the very meaning of professionalism in Western culture; a meaning which holds that ideas about good/bad, right/wrong, and appropriate/inappropriate are best established almost entirely from within the guild, from inside the circle of peers. It is this assumption of private prerogative to establish one's own ethical standards—and finally to be accountable only to peers (that is, to reflected images of oneself)—that has generated the deepest problems of medical ethics.

Ethics and Ethos

To probe this set of assumptions further, we must look at the professional ethos of physicians as this has been traditionally understood. It is this ethos which has most powerfully shaped the ethics of physicians in the past by influencing what is perceived as good or right or fitting. Ethos is the key to understanding the texture of medical professional life and the nature of its moral vision.

In the study of animals, *ethology* is the term used to describe the investigation of how an animal experiences its world and organizes its environment. It includes such things as how the animal experiences its body, locates itself in its physical setting, how it interacts with others, the range of its movements, and how it organizes the space around it. *Human ethology* must be similarly concerned with both the animal and its social and cultural environment. Cultural anthropologists use the term *ethos* to denote the moral and affective characteristics which provide a functional human environment. It is interesting, in this regard, that the earliest use of the term "ethos" signified a stall or shed in which horses stood for shelter. Our modern usage still carries a sense of the protective cultural ambiance in which persons find significance for their lives.

Ethos, in this sense, is not to be confused with the explicit belief system or world view that people hold. Rather, an ethos, as Clifford Geertz says, is "the tone, character and quality of life," or the tacit underlying attitude that is reflected in and expressed by a formal set of beliefs.[9] The world view is the picture of how things actually are for a people; the ethos is the character or tone of life which supports that picture and makes it convincing.

Formal systems of ethics express the world view, but it is the ethos which provides an ambiance in which those formal ethical views can make sense and take meaning. The professional ethos of medicine lies at the base of its ethics as a powerful set of sentiments and supporting structures. The ethical rules and principles are what are held in the formal systems of thought; the professional ethos is what is assumed. Our task here is to elicit this professional ethos and probe its assumptions.

Codes of medical ethics are but one index of the professional ethos of physicians, but they can be very revealing of basic assumptions. What is important about codes is not what they actually say, but the character of the physician which the codes accredit, and the nature of the world they portray. Generally, these codes list formulations of rules which bespeak a moral ethos severely shrunken in scope and narrow in vision. For example, the Hippocratic Oath and the larger corpus of Hippocratic writings are expressive of a primitive guild-ethics in which the primary obligations are those of doctors to their teachers and peers. The other statements are generally prohibitive rules, e.g., injunctions against seducing patients or using the knife.

The codes of the American Medical Association invest the profession with a similar kind of insularity. The AMA Code of Ethics of 1847 is largely a model for gentlemanly decorum based on Percival's *Medical Ethics* (1803). Here physicians are enjoined to "study, also, in their deportment, so as to unite tenderness with steadiness, and condescension with authority, as to inspire the minds of their patients with gratitude, respect, and confidence." The guiding assumption is that service rendered is a philanthropic gesture to patients. With some moderation in tone, this assumption still prevails in the current AMA "Principles of Medical Ethics," chiefly in the claims to physician autonomy, lack of accountability, and freedom to serve whom one chooses.

The full text of the "Principles of Medical Ethics," adopted by the House of Delegates on July 22, 1980, is as follows:

PREAMBLE: The medical profession has long subscribed to a body of ethical statements developed primarily for the benefit of the patient. As a member of this profession, a physician must recognize responsibility not only to patients, but also to society, to other health professionals, and to self. The following Principles adopted by the American Medical Association are not laws, but standards of conduct which define the essentials of honorable behavior for the physician.

I. A physician shall be dedicated to providing competent medical service with compassion and respect for human dignity.

II. A physician shall deal honestly with patients and colleagues, and strive to expose those physicians deficient in character or competence, or who engage in fraud or deception.

III. A physician shall respect the law and also recognize a responsibility to seek changes in those requirements which are contrary to the best interest of the patient.

IV. A physician shall respect the rights of patients, of colleagues, and of other health professionals, and shall safeguard patient confidences within the constraints of the law.

V. A physician shall continue to study, apply and advance scientific knowledge, make relevant information available to patients, colleagues, and the public, obtain consultation, and use the talents of other health professionals when indicated.

VI. A physician shall, in the provision of appropriate patient care, except in emergencies, be free to choose whom to serve, with whom to associate, and the environment in which to provide medical services.

VII. A physician shall recognize a responsibility to participate in activities contributing to an improved community.

The 1980 "Principles" perpetuate the tradition. This document expresses prerogatives for self-regulation, while stressing the autonomy of the individual practitioner. Patient welfare is said to be the aim and purpose of the "Principles," but only a vague sense of what this welfare might mean or how a physician might protect it is indicated. Moreover, there are a number of conspicuous omissions from the document, not the least of which are no mention of social justice in the distribution of physician services and no affirmation of the equality of patients as persons. The overall impression of the "Principles" is thereby of a union or guild ethics, a statement made by craftsmen to protect their self-interest and in which their prerogatives and rights form the central motif. The listed duties and obligations are thought to be self-imposed and freely assumed. They do not appear in any way to have been thought to be acknowledged duties based on a previous relationship of responsibility between physicians and the general public. In fact, there is no lively sense of the common good at all, except as this might be a spinoff from the good one does oneself. Rather than reflect a larger cultural tradition of ethics, the "Principles" are written as if they were the *creatio ex nihilo* of doctors. It is in this deep sense that codes of ethics within medicine have traditionally reflected an ethics fully autonomous and professionalized, and an ethos of moral sentiments severely attenuated in both scope and depth. From such a tradition of ethics and its underlying ethos have come our conventional notions of doctor-patient relationships and our accustomed ideas about the authority of physicians. It is to these considerations that we now turn.

Ethics and Authority

The authority of the physician during the greater part of the twentieth century has been sustained by a combination of powerful reciprocal assumptions. These postulates, held by patients and physicians alike, function as cultural paradigms in America for how physicians and patients understand themselves and how each understands and relates to the other. If only to begin the exploration of these cultural presuppositions, some familiar typologies may be helpful. The two which we will examine briefly are the Aesculapian authority of the physician and the patient's assumption of the sick role.

Aesculapian authority is a term coined by T. T. Paterson; but it was most fruitfully employed by Miriam Siegler and Humphrey Osmond who defined the term as a potent combination of (1) sapiential, (2) moral, and (3) charismatic authority. They further delineated these aspects of authority as correspondingly derived from (1) expertise and knowledge, (2) seeking the high value of health, and (3) God-given grace. Their analysis went on to indicate how each of these elements is traditionally associated with the physician and is, to some extent, they believe, essential to a physician's capacity to heal.[10]

Talcott Parsons's notion of the "sick role" is a good stalking horse for similar reasons; it is widely accepted by social theorists as definitive for proper patient behavior, and it is the traditional complement to Aesculapian authority. On the terms of this typology, a person becomes a patient when he or she becomes ill, is excused from normal responsibilities, places him/herself in the hands of a competent physician, and cooperates with the regimen recommended by the physician. In Parson's scheme, patients are dependent on physicians not only for therapy, but also for legitimation of their illness.[11] The sick role is thus logically the only role-set that would make the exercise of Aesculapian authority possible.

Together these typologies form a tight, interlocking notion of physician-patient encounters. The physician is active, the patient is passive; the physician is knowledgeable, the patient is ignorant; most important, the physician is authoritatve, the patient is dependent. In short, the physician-patient relationship has been dominated by a paternal image of the physician, as understood from both physician and patient perspectives. It is therefore not strange that codes of medical ethics are couched in terms of the physician's self-imposed obligations, wherein physicians are portrayed as altruistic and educated persons who, out of concern for the importunate ill, provide services to them. As true professionals, physicians have generally viewed themselves as autonomous and self-regulating, serving whom they choose, and owing first allegiance to their peers and teachers. Pellegrino, in describing this image of the physician, believes that this perception has attained a "quasi-scriptural stature."[12] Yet he and others of us share the view that this Aesculapian tradition is a troubled one.

In an insightful essay, titled "Professionalized Service and Disabling Help," John McKnight has suggested some of the reasons that service-dominated societies generally are in both economic and professional difficulty.[13] While, for example, it has been traditionally possible to decide between wheat and steel, it seems politically impossible to decide between health and education because health and education are not choices; they are services. It is, of course, the nature of a service to be something one pays for; and that something is a good which is called "care." Care, in turn, is an act that is expressive of love ("I care for her more than anyone else in the world" or "I am taking care of my family"). The resulting equation, according to McKnight, is plain: to love is to care, and care for pay is service.[14] But it is precisely the apolitical nature of service, owing to the universal value of love, which makes it virtually impossible for the public and policy makers to resolve the unprecedented politics of deciding between and among-competing services.

Further compounding this problem is another prominent symbol, "need." How need gets joined to the other rhetoric is explained by McKnight:

We say love is a need. Care is a need. Service is a need. Servicers meet needs. People are collections of needs. Society has needs. The economy should be organized to meet needs. If a need is a lack of something, to distinguish the mask from the face of service we should ask what is lacking? Some respond that we lack enough doctors, teachers, lawyers, social workers and psychiatrists. Others say that we lack enough health, knowledge, justice, social and mental well being. In a modernized society where the major business is service, the realistic political answer is that we mainly lack an adequate income for professional servicers and the economic growth they portend. The masks of love and care obscure the critical political issues of modernized societies—the necessity to manufacture needs in order to rationalize a service economy. Thus, Medicare, Educare, Judicare, Socialcare and Psychocare can be understood as systems to meet the needs of servicers and the economies they support. Removing the mask of love shows us the face of servicers who *need* income, and an economic system that *needs* growth. Within this framework, the client is less a person in need than a person who is needed. . . . The central political issue becomes the servicers' capacity to manufacture needs in order to expand the economy of the servicing system.[15]

Professionalized services thus define both the need and the service which will remedy the need; which means that if I have (or am!) a problem, the professionalized servicer is the answer. The power of the remedy to define the need, according to McKnight, is "disabling help." Indeed, there is no greater power than the authority to define the question because it enables the servicer to determine the need rather than meeting the need(s) as perceived by the client. What else has much unnecessary surgery been attributed to except an oversupply of surgeons? McKnight himself mentions an article by Birgette Berger, who suggested that baldness will soon be defined as a disease because of a surfeit of dermatologists!

The result of this professionalized progression is clear: citizens, ordinary people, neither know what they need, nor can they really understand the need or the remedy. The ordinary person's last residual hope has been at the heart of the consumer movement—we can at least assess the results of being serviced! But even this valiant last stand appears doomed. McKnight cites Thomas Dewar, whose paper ("The Professionalization of the Client") "demonstrates how the medical system is training citizens to understand that their satisfaction should be derived from being effective clients rather than people whose problem is resolved."[16] The sum of the disabling characteristics of professionalized service, according to McKnight, is thus "an ideology that converts citizens to clients, communities to deficient individuals, and politics to a self-serving debate over which service system should have a larger share of the gross national product."

Although, as we have seen, there is considerable evidence which appears to tend toward a verdict, the jury, as it were, is still out on the matter of the eventual impact of professionalized service. Meantime, two factors—cultural pluralism and egalitarianism—serve increasingly to erode Aesculapian authority and the conventional sick role. Cultural pluralism is so much a fact of contemporary America that it affects every institution, large and small, including medicine. So completely is pluralism regnant in this society that diversity of lifestyles and values is now virtually taken for granted. Functionally, pluralism is individualism in multilateral relationships. It is therefore not surprising that existence as a distinct, separate entity (i.e., an individual) has come to be exalted as a positive virtue—which may explain, at least in part, why we more often refer to ourselves as a "society" (a colony of organisms) than as a "community" (a social group which shares common interests).

Withal, the diversity of which we speak is pervasive and extends to the value(s) of health and the role(s) of the physician. It is thus little wonder that patients no longer automatically assume the characteristics of the sick role, or that there are increasing professionally managed service systems which are attempting to deal with this remnant of resistance! Indeed, even the very definitions of sickness are being altered. One million unruly school children are annually given Ritalin and other amphetamines even though there are only 100,000 clinically diagnosed cases of hyperkinesis in the country, and homosexuality is no longer officially classified as an illness; changes which are accountable not only to pupil-management problems in the schools and gay rights activism, but also to the incipient variability of definitions of illness in a pluralistic society.

More generally, the assumed consonance between physician and patient values has been replaced by divergence and occasional conflict of values. Every doctor must sometime experience the resistance, anger, and hostility of a patient. In fact, we have observed, even in consultations involving a high-technology "innovative therapy," which offers to patients in extremis with chronic disease syndromes just a thread of undemonstrated hope, that these patients customarily tend to express an adversarial attitude toward the physician. In sum, diversity has become perversity inasmuch as there is little (or, at best, insufficient) commonality between and among us; the ethos of community has buckled under the weight of individualism and its social expression in pluralism.

A second major force which has diminished traditional physician authority is the egalitarian push toward altering power discrepancies in almost every dimension of social and political relationships. Many patients now demand to participate in decisions which affect them, and thereby seek collaborative associations with physicians. Valid consent—and, on the negative side, malpractice suits—are symbols of patients' desire for power of information, or redress of grievances, in order to strengthen and establish the patient role vis-à-vis physicians. Medical power that was formerly seen as beneficial is now sometimes seen as arbitrary and oppressive; the dependency features of the sick role are no longer attractive or tolerable. And the result is that the authority of Aesculapius, which was treasured *by patients* as a curative power in the past, is now frequently viewed as capricious and unjustified power—a usurpation of patient prerogatives.

A good example of this shift in physician paradigms, away from the paternal care model, can be seen in the current debate over truth-telling. The traditional assumptions are nicely reflected in the American Medical Association Judicial Council's *Opinions and Reports,* which carries the following statement under the heading, "Prognosis": "The physician should neither exaggerate nor minimize the gravity of a patient's condition. He should assure himself that the patient, his relatives or his responsible friends have such knowledge of the patient's condition as will serve the best interests of the patient and the family."[17]

Our purpose here is not to repudiate this maxim but to show how it reflects a traditional ethics based on the assumptions of Aesculapian prerogatives. It is, to be sure, commendable to have the best interests of the patient and the family in clear and prominent focus. But the axial issue is: whose notion of "best" is the appropriate one? And on what value predicates does that notion rest? The Aesculapian physician presumes to make this decision as a matter of professional competence; indeed, the Aesculapian physician believes that he holds this power as a trust and an obligation of superior knowledge, experience, and expertise. Thus, relating a diagnosis—or whether to disclose it at all—is thought to be a privilege entirely within the professional's discretion.

It is not simply that physicians are thought to know more than others regarding the diagnosis, or that they should know best how to communicate what they know; in the Aesculapian tradition, that knowledge is presumed to warrant a moral corollary, namely that professional knowledge of diagnosis is also knowledge of what is *good for* the patient. Sapiential authority is thereby backed by moral authority; they become mutually reinforcing. And it is precisely at this juncture that physicians have been recently challenged. The major critics of medicine have not challenged doctors on epistemic grounds—what they know, or how they presume to know it; rather these critics have demurred at the use of that knowledge in terms of the moral legitimacy of the agent who wields knowledge. Their question is, "How can the patient be assured that the physician will seek *his or her* good rather than some good rooted in the physician's values?"

This should not be a surprising query, if only because the situations in which physicians can exercise the power of defining "the good" are numerous. Persons suffering from heart disease are often told that they "ought" to change their eating habits and lifestyle. Males with hypertension are frequently encouraged to think that they "should" sacrifice potency for the promise of longevity. Pediatricians sometimes put it to the parents of a deformed newborn that they "must" radically alter their lives to accommodate this biological tragedy. On the other hand, patients are now frequently saying that what is medically best and what is humanly and personally best may conflict; that the coincidence of these two, when it happens, is a gracious event but not the foregone conclusion upon entering a clinic or a working premise of their consent to medical intervention.

The most potent and pervasive professional power is the authority to define what is good, for it is on this cornerstone prerogative that the other authorities of the Aesculapian physician are built. It is an assumption of the Aesculapian tradition that this authority belongs naturally to the physician. This is not only because of the high value placed on health but it is due, more subtly, to the conflation of goodness with knowledge which the physician is perceived to possess. To see this connection more clearly we need to return to Francis Bacon.

"The Good" Masked by
Professional Knowledge

There are chiefly two ways in which Bacon's empirical experimental method has had profound impact on modernity. First of all, from Bacon's definition of what is knowable we are reduced to the claim that we can possess knowledge of nature but that we emphatically do not possess knowledge of ourselves, of our own "human nature," and of those institutions and cultures and concerns which lie closest to us as human beings. There is a natural objectivity, but a human subjectivity; there is an unspanned gulf between nature and spirit, between what is called science and what is called wisdom. Or, to put the matter somewhat differently, Bacon's methodology sunders fact and value. That alone is a very serious matter for the reason that it bifurcates human culture, both by making the only profitable avenue to truth-finding the experimental method, and by making art, history, politics, ethics, and other fields of humanistic knowledge either useless or dubious. So a certain authority attaches to "nature" as it is scientifically understood and explained, alongside which any other human authority is denigrated and compelled to submission.

This leads to the second way in which Bacon's legacy has enormously influenced us: Bacon's disciples in the social sciences proceeded to reduce the explicitly human to the realm of nature. By the application of the experimental method to human phenomena, the subject was objectified quite as nature had been. The "Thou" was rendered into an "it." From Condorcet through the British empiricists (Hartley, Priestly, Bentham) the notion of determinism was developed—that is, through education or propaganda or law, men and women could be conditioned to become whatever the superordinate authority desired them to become. And with Auguste Comte, the reduction of man to automaton received its clearest advocacy: it is the business of sociology, Comte claimed, to learn the laws of social phenomena and then apply them to make "the Great Being." Thereafter it only remained to Marxism (and other repressive political systems, as well) to exploit the political possibilities of this approach: man is what he may become through the scientific knowledge of man, and through manipulation by those who know the social laws. Marxism and totalitarianism are the practical outworkings of the Baconian thesis.

Bacon deliberately restricted the range of knowledge in order to gain increased control, and by excluding the whole area of what we have called "wisdom" he made knowledge more certain; but that benefit was achieved at the cost of comprehensiveness and significance. In Bacon's view, knowledge is power; but he only *assumed* that what he knew and controlled was *good* because value questions, why a thing is good, were specifically excluded by his utilitarianism.

It has been our legacy since the time of Bacon to denigrate value hypotheses which are not, or have not been, or cannot be, derived from scientific positivism. That tendency has marked the ascendancy of *techne* over *philosophia* and the subordination of wisdom to technics. But it has not always been so in Western culture. Another ancient argued that knowledge in the highest sense is not technics (in the modern sense of that word). According to Plato, information without enlightenment is as good as, or worse than, nothing. Indeed, technical knowledge, which Protagoras said was the gift of Prometheus to man, was no guarantee at all against ignorance of the worst sort. This is so, Plato argued, because the sciences (arithmetic, geometry, astronomy) are helpful propaedeutic studies—that is, they facilitate and indeed liberate the understanding from mere sensationalism. But the "learning" afforded by science is not yet formed by "knowledge"; and for Plato it was knowledge which complements information with moral earnestness.

Students on surgical rounds were puzzled by a patient admitted with repeat gastric ulcer, until the attending surgeon reminded them that the two most common causes of this condition were domestic and employment anxieties; whereupon the students belatedly inquired and "discovered" that this patient was unemployed, deeply in debt, and his wife chronically ill! By "moral earnestness" Plato meant that without virtue and love the information which science offers us is undirected, anomic, and avails us nothing in pursuit of the good. The sciences, as explorations in sensation, incur many private worlds but have no way to escape from "solitary assertion" and thus have no knowledge which is communicable (i.e., corroborative) and articulate (i.e., shared) by a community of kindred minds. In a word, these data are not responsible or accountable. They may be true opinion (*doxa alethes*) which is valid; but, according to Plato, knowledge requires more than private surmise: it must be jointly acknowledged and possessed in common in order to be truly knowledge.

The objectivist theory of truth attempts to present a picture of reality in which any personal attribution, and especially from the person presenting the picture, is absent. But the error of that theory is precisely that the human factor cannot be excluded. There are no uninterpreted facts; it is a particular scientist's judgment, experience, knowledge, intuition, and all the rest which play an indispensable role in marking a given contribution to knowledge as having been made by this person and no other. So it was Benjamin Duggar, and no other, who discovered aureomycin; Wilhelm Roentgen, and no other, who is credited with discovering x-rays; William Harvey, and no other, whose breakthroughs in studying the heart and circulation are still celebrated; Christiaan Barnard, and no other, who performed the first human cardiac homograft; and on and on the list would go.

The scientist, in short, is a man or a woman who does not cease to be a man or a woman by virtue of lab coat, or test tubes, or microscope, or whatever other paraphernalia attend the role of scientist. We believe that it is important for both scientists and nonscientists to recognize and remember that elemental fact.

The sum of the matter is that there is no achievement of knowledge, by whatever method, which is not conditioned by a prior human decision about what is worth knowing; that is, what it is good to know, why we ought to know it, and what we intend to do with it once we have acquired that knowledge. And it is for this fairly obvious and commonplace reason that knowledge is not disinterested, but value-preferenced, from the start. Wisdom consists of both cognitive and axiological aspects. That is similarly why Bacon's purposes for the experimental method are neither objective nor immutable; they rest on a certain human view of how things are and how things ought to be, and they are therefore powerless except as we grant them power. It should be no cause for wonder, then, that people should question what is medically best and what is humanly and personally best. "Being healthy" and "being human" rest upon human predications of meaning and value which, depending upon how they are viewed, assert their complementarity or their antagonism.

In summary, the ethos of scientific methodology has produced a sort of amnesia about values within us. We commonly neglect the way in which knowledge is in the service of some good, real or imagined. The knowledge held and exercised by professionals is especially so value-laden, yet the deference we pay to medical professionals serves to obscure these value dimensions. These assumptions about what is good are masked by the assumed beneficence of knowledge and the desirability of professional services and goals. Coupled with the traditional insularity of professional norms, these forces serve as a barrier to the critical review of ethics in medicine. Hence, there is need to probe for moral values, not only within individual physician judgments but also within the ethos which undergirds individual judgments. There is furthermore need to ask, at tacit and explicit levels, at individual and social levels, within professions and for the larger culture, about all of our assumed values, "But what is good?"

But What Is Good?

Medical intervention currently rests upon two precursory premises; one of which is quite explicit but the other of which is tacit, and to this point largely unexamined and unacknowledged by either professionals or the lay public. The explicit premise consists of all those ways in which human life is thought to benefit from, or be improved upon, or served by medical intervention. On this premise, which is clearly affirmed in scientific medicine together with most of the literature of medical ethics, we have proceeded with the development of *in utero* diagnosis, ectogenesis, coronary artery bypass, and the like— that is, with all those techniques which are supposed to be remedies or therapies for some human problem.

But the unexamined and tacit presupposition is that human life can and ought to be improved upon, or made better in discrete ways, by these kinds of interventions. To talk about "improving" or "bettering" is, of course, to introduce a *genre* of considerations which involves value categories and, by definition, embraces the public whose "betterment" or "improvement" is envisioned.

Our experience, both here and in Europe, is that scientists, physicians, economists, sociologists, and others increasingly share the view that interdisciplinary and interprofessional colleagueship is both necessary and possible, especially for clarification of the values associated with this work. And congruent with this view is another which is gaining acknowledgment: that policy formation demands the varied points of view of many competencies, not the least of which are the perspectives of patients.

Three questions, in particular, emerge from the tacit dimension of medical intervention: (*a*) *who* has authority to make these decisions for "betterment" or "improvement," and what credentials are fitting for those who would make these judgments? (*b*) *why* are these interventions "good," that is, what are the moral predicates upon which these decisions might be taken; in other words *how,* in what way, is our circumstance "better" with than without these interventions? and (*c*) *what* assurance or guarantee or promise or hope do we reasonably have that these interventions will produce happier or healthier or better people, or more human societies, or a larger measure of justice, or whatever is supposed under the canons of humane sensibility to be a desirable goal?

Suspicious of professional definitions of "good" and "beneficial" and "better," fearing them to be self-serving, skeptical of notions of the "common good" and apprehensive that they are provincial, patients now frequently seek to be empowered to speak for themselves. Our point is not that the statement on prognosis by the Judicial Council is somehow wrong; at issue are the grounds for distinguishing right from wrong—who most appropriately does this, and on what predicates? Meantime, the Aesculapian tradition is heavily vested in the professional autonomy of the physician which, by definition, leaves little room for any kind of fiduciary, cooperative, covenanting relationship with the patient. (The converse situation, in which patient autonomy dominates, clearly would not resolve this problem. But why patient autonomy is so obviously intolerable ought itself to be highly suggestive to the moral imagination of those who fail to view the Aesculapian tradition as at all problematic.)

Aesculapian authority has become morally ambiguous. It may be seen as beneficent protection, or as the exercise of raw power; but both of these views are grounded in a set of assumptions about professionals, and particularly physicians, which are no longer commonly held. The ethics of physicians, when so conceived, may surely be undergirded by the professionalized ethos; but it is not any longer popularly endorsed by the public at large. For all these reasons, new formulations of physician authority are required.

3 ◇ Moral Imagination and Medicine

Moral Imagination

Michael Novak has said that "the main force shaping our symbolic world today is professionalism—the expert in the white coat, his peers watching him, his techniques polished, his mind 'tough,' his knowledge 'hard.' If we wish to break out of that captivity, we must attack it in its stronghold; its grip over our imagination, over our sense of reality, and over our institutions."[1] Medicine is clearly the paradigm which Novak had in mind. And our previous arguments about professional ethics, and the ethos which supports it, are meant to probe precisely these matters. Our contention is not that doctors have had insufficient or inaccurate principles to guide their practice of medicine; still less have we wanted to imply that doctors are somehow motivated by wrong intentions and self-serving ends. Both of these are only surface, superficial conclusions. The problem of professional ethics in medicine lies, we think, at the level of ethological assumptions, that is, with the largely unexamined figures and metaphors which animate the moral imagination of physicians (and, to some extent, patients as well).

Physicians are not alone, as we have pointed out, in their loyalty to quite conventional scenarios of "the good"; other professional groups are similarly committed to and motivated by them. But that may not be the most striking dimension of professional ethics in the present situation. It is surely true that professionals still insist upon, and like to think of themselves as, being self-defined and self-regulating; but in a *service* profession, it is also essential to appreciate the ways in which professionals themselves are not solely responsible for how their moral imagination gets shaped. The environing society irreducibly participates in this process. It is obvious that physicians are part of American culture, and it is probably just as obvious that physicians share with the larger public many basic norms and values. It may not, however, be quite so obvious how physician values are formed in many ways by the requirements which patients place upon them; or how physician values reflect the lay public's norms for what the doctor "should" be and do.

Mass media, for example, played a very important role in cardiac transplantation in the period immediately following Christiaan Barnard's initial attempts. The press, together with radio and television, celebrated Barnard's first two procedures (December 3 and 6, 1967) and described the surgery as "heart transplant success" and "the ultimate operation." Indeed, television crews were admitted to Barnard's operating theater; and almost instantaneously he was lionized (and later other prominent cardiovascular surgeons) on TV screens throughout the world. One result of this immediate notoriety was an enormous pressure, exerted on surgeons by a desperate but hopeful public that was itself sometimes misled by euphoric and incorrect reporting, to perform heart transplants. The consequence, as we now know, was that some transplantation was done under less than optimal circumstances by less than adequately staffed and trained teams on patients who were at inordinate risk. Moreover, certain breaches occurred in the conventional code of professional conduct as some surgeons seized the potential value of media exposure for facility and research funds, for potential donors and recipients, as well as for gaining the upper hand in some intramural professional quarrels. The role of mass and instantaneous media, as part of ethical assessment, has been too long and too much neglected; all the same, its deportment in the early history of cardiac homografting is instructive regarding the vulnerability of physicians to others' expectations of them.

The value system of American culture has a lofty place for experts and schools us in an excessive dependence upon them. Utopian expectations of health and well-being tend to keep health professionals at a safe remove from our usual expectations of failure, while simultaneously these same expectations equip us to be hypercritical when errors do occur (or even when outcomes are less than optimal). We are an overmedicalized society in large part because we have committed so many of our expectations for "the good life" to medical intervention, and correspondingly abdicated large responsibility for our own health. We engage in sexual intercourse without appropriate contraceptive precaution because abortion is available to solve the problem of unwanted pregnancy; or we do not exercise and ingest diets high in cholesterols and triglycerides without too much worry about coronary artery disease because surgical transplant and bypass procedures are available; or we drive automobiles under the influence of alcohol, or ride motorcycles without protective clothing and helmets, or never bother with seatbelts and harnesses in the hope that head trauma units await us in most emergency rooms. Our task therefore cannot be a repudiation of physician norms so much as it is an effort to describe a public and professional ethos—supported by physicians and laypersons alike—which no longer serves the larger goals of either doctor or patient, or the common good.

We argued earlier that Western culture has tended over the last three centuries toward egalitarianism and individualism; in view of that, our current claim—that we rely too heavily on experts of all sorts—may sound strange. If these two assertions are logically contradictory, they are not experientially so. Patients can assume the sick role because they believe that they will receive better care and, at the same time, deeply resent the fact that they feel constrained to assume that role as a condition of receiving good care. What is otherwise and customarily most cherished—namely, staunch individualism and egalitarian sentiment—seems (naturally?!) to give way to excessive dependence and personal anonymity when we fall ill. What is missing, of course, is some sense of mutual interdependence and personal collaboration between doctors and patients; but this will be possible only in conjunction with some different sense of *why* patients come to see physicians and *on what basis* physicians respond to medically defined human distress.

The Samaritan Paradigm

The moral imagination of physicians is traditionally populated with figures of individuals performing heroic acts of supererogation—something like what is portrayed in the story of the Good Samaritan. That parable goes like this:

A man was going down from Jerusalem to Jericho, and fell among robbers who stripped him and beat him, and departed leaving him half dead. Now by chance a priest was going down that road, and when he saw him he passed by on the other side. So likewise a Levite, when he came to the place and saw him passed by on the other side. But a Samaritan, as he journeyed, came where he was; and when he saw him he had compassion. And went to him and bound up his wounds, pouring on oil and wine, and set him on his own beast and brought him to an inn, and took care of him. And the next day he took out two denarii and gave them to the innkeeper, saying, "Take care of him; and whatever more you spend, I will repay you when I come back."[2]

There are many aspects, some of them very subtle, which attend this story; but our interest here is restricted to the rather obvious ways in which the story is generally regarded as a moving one, and a worthy paradigm for virtuous action. The Samaritan goes out of his way, at some cost to himself, to provide help for a perfect stranger who is in need. Instead of being treated as a parable, the story is sometimes esteemed as a moral norm. But problems arise when the-story-as-moral-norm is taken to exhaust the nature of moral obligation. As Judith Jarvis Thomson has pointed out, the heroic character of the Samaritan's action overshadows the sense of minimal decency which one should have been able to expect from the priest and the Levite![3] And when that happens, the model for virtue is not "minimal decency," but "good Samaritanism" or even "supererogatory Samaritanism"—that is, an isolated individual act which is distinguished by heroic proportions of splendor and largesse. Such acts, when they happen, are truly magnificent and bound to capture attention. But with professionals, minimum levels of moral obligation, in the long run of routine practice, may be more important than high ideals. This is because most moral problems have to do, not with the lack of altitude and amplitude of moral ideals, but with the breadth and depth of a vision of "the good" which permits us to employ our high ideals in routine situations.

Raymond Duff put it succinctly when he said that the "aspirational heroism" which has frequently motivated the professional must share its place with "humble heroism."[4] Aspirational heroism trades upon the romantic image of the health professional as always saving lives through extraordinary feats of skill—snatching patients literally from the jaws of death (and the doctor, incidentally, from defeat). Power, skill, and conquest of nature through empirical experimental knowledge are cardinal virtues of the aspirational hero. The humble hero, on the other hand, achieves somewhat different sorts of victories; not always over disease or nature, but by exercising dominion over the debilitating aspects of illness and death, namely abandonment, anxiety, loss of control, and pain. Virtuous professionalism here is no

longer prowess in knowledge and technical skill or victory over
death, but steadfastness, loyalty, and fidelity to patients and their
families.

A physician friend has suggested that it is important to ask, Who
are the real heroes in medicine and surgery? The names which recur
time and again in the literature are those of the surgeons who head
transplant teams or the physicians who demonstrate the efficacy of
some drug; when the names of patients (or subjects) occur, it is
chiefly for the purpose of identifying a particular incident. Our friend
thinks that the real heroes may be those patients and subjects who
put themselves, their bodies and lives, on the line; and he wonders
why, in this transaction, the ones with least to lose are the ones who
gain the most in terms of recognition and praise. Who remembers
the names of Barnard's first two cardiac homograft recipients, or of
the first recipient in the United States? On another front, who remembers the name of the first U.S. astronaut? Publicity associated
with the space programs, in both the United States and the USSR,
poses a novel alternative: the heroes celebrated in these technical
triumphs *are* the astronauts, whose encapsulated relationship with
earthbound support groups may not, in the final analysis, be very
different from that of an anesthetized patient on an operating table
or a patient in bondage to a disease and harnessed to dependency in
a consulting room. The Good Samaritan ideal plays upon our sense
of concern for the less fortunate but it does not, as customarily interpreted, evoke our sense of interdependence and conviviality with the
person who lies beaten on the road.

We are not told whether the robber's victim gave his consent to
the Samaritan's assistance; and it may be important to consider why
this detail might have been omitted, as we try to understand other
details which were included. Acts of supererogation need no consent;
indeed, the very conditions which make an action supererogatory
also make the conventional consent requirement trivial and out-of-
place. That is why patients who come to physicians in the "sick role"
may be perceived as in such distress that a formal consent, in turn, is
thought to be superfluous or demeaning. If medicine is armed with
the moral authority of "Good Samaritanism," there is no need to
inquire about permission or appropriateness of treatment. Patients
perceived as sick and vulnerable are not supposed to be capable of
collaborative relationships. From the patient's point of view, because
these acts of assistance and healing are gratuitous, it seems indecorous

and graceless to question them. One does not ask a drowning man whether he wishes to be rescued; nor does a drowning man ask for the certified qualifications of his would-be rescuer. The metaphor of rescue, extended to large provinces of patient care, remains a major image which shapes physician ethics.

We reiterate that our purpose here is not to suggest that the story of the Good Samaritan is a faulty moral guide; we mean simply to point out that, when translated into the American imagination and placed within the ethos of medicine, the message of the story tends to look like philanthropy. What usually goes unnoticed in our appropriation of this story is that the Samaritan acts out of compassion. He does not act out of altruism or *noblesse oblige,* nor does he see his help as fulfillment of a duty or an ideal or even a free and noble act. We are told, rather, that he is *moved by compassion* upon seeing the man in the road. Compassion means literally "to feel with," and denotes a sense of identification and community.[5] Compassion is not saccharine pity or demeaning self-righteousness to the less fortunate; neither is it associated with the charisma which forms part of the physician's traditional authority. Indeed, it is precisely these misconstruals which are offensive and insulting to the sick. Authentic compassion, on the other hand, engages one genuinely and empathetically in community with another.

Doubtless one of the reasons that compassion is overlooked in our usual reading of the Samaritan paradigm is that the ideal professional is ordinarily characterized as fully in control of his or her emotions. That control is sometimes expressed in the phrase, "detached concern," which conveys the idea that professionals (and, in our case, physicians) must keep a certain distance between themselves and those they care for. Various cognates—"disinterested sympathy," "affective neutrality," "detachment"—are employed to express the same idea. All of these terms point to the professional distance which is believed to be necessary for the achievement of therapeutic goals, and all of them are supposed to be indispensable for objectivity. Their overall impact limits the personal (i.e., nonprofessional) involvement of the physician with the patient, thereby protecting both parties and preserving good judgment while prohibiting judgmental attitudes.

But detachment as the preeminent criterion of professional style has always been inadequate; and in a pluralistic culture, it is genuinely detrimental. Alternatively, the affective dimension is one of the most fecund of human capacities, and it is the real presupposition for more formal knowledge of patients. It is, then, not simply good bedside manner to know the patient; it is good medicine, because the ability to feel what the patient feels is that "minimal sense of decency" which makes appropriate intervention permitted. Compassion is the highest form of affective acuity, and is therefore a skill to be cultivated because it is a moral requirement for effective practice. In this sense, compassion is not merely a feeling; it is a moral sense, a way of relating to others which accredits their humanity and confirms one's own to them, and in that process connects these two in com-unity.

Professional Ethics Reconsidered

Primary care medicine is, in many ways, a significant departure from the professionalized traditions which we have been examining. In the first chapter, we reviewed some common understandings of primary care; now here, as there, our purpose is not to achieve a definitive statement but to gather some ideas that cluster around primary care and begin to assess their meaning. Because primary care is not just a new label for traditional medicine but a new way of practicing medicine, new ways of being "professional" are entailed, with novel sources for authority, and different criteria for the use of power. In brief, primary care entails a new understanding of professional ethics because it is symbolic of a different cultural ethos within which this kind of professional ethics can function.

Whatever definition of primary care one espouses, some notions are fairly constant. Among these are an emphasis on the patient as a psychosocial being as well as an instance of a disease entity, and the assumption of a larger and consistent responsibility for patient care over time—in contradistinction, we can say, to the episodic and discontinuous patterns which currently prevail in secondary and tertiary care. On the face of it, these ideas do not sound like radical departures from traditional medicine; but on closer examination they are antithetical to the prevailing standards of professionalized ethics. The notions surrounding primary care bespeak a different ethos; they suggest a different source for the physician's authority to treat, as well as a new scope of accountability; they necessitate a relationship with patients which is more collaborative than paternal, more mutual than unilateral. Many, perhaps even most, physicians would ascribe to these goals and want to deliver this kind of care; but that is made difficult by the traditionally professionalized ethics which narrowly defines the terms of work and carefully guards the autonomy of practitioners.

The definitions of primary care also stipulate alternative forms of practice, not just as common sense but as responsibilities of the practitioner. For example, the Institute of Medicine study insists that accessibility is a *conditio sine qua non* for primary care. By this term the authors denote availability, attainability, and acceptability.[6] Accessibility, in this context, means not only temporal availability when needed and attainability in terms of the cost of services; it also means acceptability of services to patients. Put plainly, professional services must be offered in terms commensurate with the patient's sense of what those services are and how they can be used. Thus, psychological and social elements complement professional accessibility. This is clearly a basic condition for any good practice, but the primary care ideal makes it explicit and even goes a step beyond. The primary care model portrays a condition for the initial rendering of care which shapes the continuing doctor-patient relationship. Moreover, it is the very opposite of the idea of noblesse oblige as it suggests that the physician should maintain a practice based upon the social and cultural realities of his or her patient population.

What does all this do to the traditional ideal of Aesculapian authority? It subverts it entirely. Aesculapian authority holds that authority is derived from the status of knowledge and the inherent good of the role—that is, the differentiated behavior of physicians. Doctors possess authority simply by being doctors. Because of their knowledge, because they seek noble goals and socially desired ends, they are given authority to treat. So the Aesculapian portrait of authority goes. By invoking criteria of acceptability, however, primary care definitions lodge the authority of physicians not in the office or social position or knowledge, but in the ability of physicians to meet patient needs. That is again why primary care bespeaks not a new specialty but a new way of practicing medicine; that is also why the definitions of primary care offer ways to rethink medical ethics. In order to explore the critical dimensions of that rethinking, we can examine briefly the patient's interpretation of illness and the meaning of valid consent.

Models of Illness

It will come as no surprise to anyone who has observed physicians and patients together that patients' ideas about their sickness are often quite different from physicians' understandings of illness and disease. Indeed, beyond the obvious discrepancies of expertise, training, and professional preoccupation, there are more subtle differences which tend to distance patients from physicians, and vice versa. It is important, in order to illuminate some of this subtlety, that we distinguish between the conventional medical model and what we have observed to be a fairly customary model which patients adopt. We emphatically do not mean to imply that these models are static structures, or even archetypes; instead, we use the metaphor of models to denote differences in patient and professional expectations, values, and perceptions. These models, in turn, become morally significant inasmuch as they help to shape our sense of what is thought, by the parties involved, to be "right," or "good," or "appropriate."

The medical model is commonly taken to be a biomedical view of reality which assumes that, in the understanding and treatment of illness, organic concerns are more basic, "real," clinically significant, and worthy of attention than any other set of data. The medical model thus, on its own terms, reasonably transforms a patient's illness into a disease which is a recognizable entity in the Western classificatory system. This is not to say that the medical model necessarily treats human beings as only bodies or like machines, or that it must view treatment as nothing more than a technological fix. All the same, the medical model does have strong perceptual biases, together with correlative language structures, which make mechanistic interpretation and technological solution attractive. In its typical progression, the medical model is concerned with such items as onset of symptoms, disease etiology, pathophysiology, natural history of the disease, and potential for treatment via intervention.

In somewhat striking contrast, the patient model is ordinarily concerned with the meaning of the illness. Social and anthropological studies have consistently shown that patient compliance and satisfaction—as well as responses to pain, frequency of use of the health care system, and the like—are related to important social phenomena like cultural tradition, occupation, social class, education, and religious belief. While only the most provincial should be surprised at these findings, social scientists have nevertheless given too-infrequent attention to the idiosyncratic detail of any particular patient's model of his or her illness; with the result of inappropriately broad generalization and stereotyping. The knowledge, for example, that patients of Irish descent tend to ignore pain, and disregard it as a symptom, may be helpful; but it is surely not definitive for any given Irishman whom one might encounter in the clinic. Crude categorizations conceal the fine texture of detail which makes up any particular patient's model of his or her illness; yet it is precisely this detail, so constitutive of the meaning of the illness for the patient, which is foreign to the medical model and thus seemingly bizarre to many health professionals.

Michel Foucault has expressed the traditional professional disregard of this detail quite well when, speaking of the beginnings of pathological anatomy in the eighteenth century, he identifies a conceptional transformation which "gave to the clinical field a new structure in which the individual in question was not so much a sick person as the endlessly reproducible pathological fact to be found in all patients suffering in a similar way."[7]

In the medical model there is not only a tendency to ignore details of a certain sort; there is the positive obligation to disregard details which are (merely!) peculiar to *this* patient because those details, *ab initio,* are really not helpful in either diagnosis or treatment. It is owing principally to the medical model that the detail of a particular patient's model for his or her illness may appear not only irrelevant but plainly unwonted to a physician. Why this is so can be laid to many reasons, but our purpose here is not to explore the origins of these interpretations; our aim, instead, is to exhibit the divergence between medical and patient models, and thereby display the moral significance of these differences.

Consider the following case. A 43-year-old college professor with chest pain was diagnosed as having angina based on coronary artery disease, but he refused to accept the diagnosis. He insisted that his physician agree to a diagnosis of pulmonary embolus. Deeper probing uncovered a widespread, but erroneous explanatory model: the belief, shared by wife and family, that angina signals the end of an active life and the beginning of invalidism. The patient therefore needed to prove that his doctor was mistaken. After eliciting the patient's model, the doctor and patient could discuss these fears, work for acceptance of the disease, and plan realistically for a course of treatment.[8]

By accrediting the psychosocial aspects of illness, primary care medicine goes a long way toward accrediting the patient's model of his or her illness. By emphasizing the acceptability of services offered to the patient, the philosophy of primary care obliges the physician at least to appreciate the patient's model as a credible factor which influences the overall effectiveness of therapy. In the case above this appreciation alleviated fears and allowed for accurate and frank discussion.

One of the more than casually interesting items sometimes found in a patient's model of illness is the belief that the cause of the illness is related to moral transgression. The patient's complete etiology may contain notions of retribution from God for previous sins, or the need for atonement and suffering for wrongdoing, whether real or imagined. Patients who suffer from cancer of the face, genitalia, or another highly valued part of the body seem especially prone to an etiology in which the illness symbolizes amends for such things as excessive vanity or infidelity to a spouse. Insistence that such notions of causality are irrational is quite beside the point since a patient's interpretation is rarely grounded in rational logic; instead, patient models cluster around questions of the personal meaning of the disease. These notions are therefore not irrational, but nonrational.

In a similar way, patient ideas about treatment differ markedly from what the physician recommends. It is no secret that a large segment of the patient population relies on multiple healing systems, and that Western medical practitioners are frequently augmented by herbalists, faith healers, self-help systems, and others whose model of illness seems to the patient to coincide more closely with the patient's own model. Cancer patients are known sometimes to detour to Vitamin C or laetrile, not simply because of fear and desperation but because these remedies are frequently presented in a way which is compelling within the patient's model of illness. In a word, these other remedies seem more "real." In this connection, it is worth noting that drug therapy is frequently compromised by patient neglect or rejection. Only 50 percent of patients take the first dose of prescribed drug regimens, and more than half of the remaining 50 percent fail to finish the full course. These behaviors become all the more striking when it is appreciated that approximately seventeen billions of dollars are spent annually in the United States for drugs, and that about 1.5 billion outpatient prescriptions were filled in 1979.[9]

The divergence between medical and patient models is sometimes of little or no moral consequence; frequently, however, the variation becomes morally problematic. Although the precise way in which moral difficulties arise from such divergence is intricate to trace, it is generally the case that there is a high risk of moral dispute when the physician insists on holding exclusively to the medical model and is thereby rendered unable to understand or empathize with the patient's interpretation. Questions of "whose understanding of the illness takes precedence" and "how treatment can or should be carried out" are examples of moral conflicts which are formed out of the clash between divergent interpretations of an illness. The incongruence between the medical model and the patient's idiosyncratic model of illness influences the quality of care, effectiveness of treatment, and recognition and ability to deal with psychosocial problems.

Many have argued persuasively that the physician must understand the psychological, social, and economic factors which influence the health of their patients; and we agree that this is obvious, commonsensical, and unarguable. But that obligation is not the claim we mean to assert here. We contend, rather, that primary care medicine implies a form of practice and an exercise of imagination such that patients' interpretive grids for their own illnesses are given due regard, and even legitimation, in the mode of the relationship established between doctor and patient. In other words, primary care implies that human and interpretive skills of relation must precede and shape the exercise of technical and biomedical skills of intervention, and extend to decisions about which therapies are appropriate.

To argue that the physician simply needs to understand social and psychological factors in illness betrays a facile view. Talking that way seeks to make the physician an amateur social scientist who "factors in" the ethnic, social, and other aspects of patients like additional pieces of diagnostic information. No doubt, if one could do this, it would be useful. Even so, such an understanding neglects the patient's own understanding of the meaning of these factors and proposes, yet again, to impose Aesculapian authority upon the physician-patient relationship. Primary care implies that understanding and acknowledging the patient's model for his or her illness is prerequisite for giving care. Our point here, if difficult to grant, is a simple one to put forward: no social scientific assessment of "factors" can approximate, much less substitute for, a patient's understanding of his or her own illness. The condition on which technical care can be assented to by the patient, and thus begin to be efficacious in the larger healing process, rests upon that understanding.

In conversation with medical colleagues, we have encountered objections at this juncture which raise the specter of emergency room resuscitation, with the standard comment: "When I am wheeled into the emergency room in cardiac arrest, I had rather have a cold and unfeeling technician who can revive me than a humanistic physician who can relate my demise to my relatives with great feeling and sensitivity!" We believe that the emergency room paradigm serves the emergency room situation well, but we reject a facsimile of the ER as appropriate for primary care. It is similarly not necessary, under usual circumstances, to choose between the brusque but efficient technician and the sensitive but incompetent doctor. The emergency is a special case with its own norms and, by definition, lacks the ordinary relational space which we think customarily appropriate between doctors and patients. Indeed, the very term "emergency" means to communicate a situation in which discretionary range and time for careful weighing of options are absent, that work is done under considerable stress, that routine amenities are suspended. Similar conditions are associated with *triage*. But in most instances the boundaries of application are set by the exceptional circumstances which define "emergency" and "triage" and within which physicians must function. That emergency rooms are used as primary care centers by some segments of the population indicates another kind of problem which the emerging definitions of primary care are meant to address.

The crux of our argument, therefore, is that the patient's model of illness cannot be reduced to the thin veneer of "psychosocial factors," but that this model bespeaks the patient as a person in time, with rituals of meaning, symbols of interpretation, and senses of self already fully developed and operating in and through the presenting illness. Although physicians can dispel unwarranted fears, they cannot, nor should they, hope to change these things substantially; they must ultimately work within the structures of meaning which the patient brings. This is the meaning of "acceptability" of services, and it is a moral requirement embedded in both the science and the art of medicine.

"Rights" as a Relational Category

Our emphasis on the acceptability of medical services to patients is not, however, a pliant endorsement of the "patients rights" position. Indeed, recourse to "rights" language, together with the litany of rights frequently cited, is as problematic as paternalistic authority. So, for example, when breasts are augmented, and noses reduced, and faces lifted, doctors may be responding to patient *desires* but hardly to a basic right to be treated for illness. Distinctions between cosmetic and reconstructive surgeries are important, and need to be further refined; but even now they suggest that cosmetic intervention is not treatment for an illness. Our emphasis on the patient's interpretation of illness is not intended and cannot be extended to cover cosmetic procedures. Likewise, tranquilizers for the nervous teenager prior to her first violin recital are not treatment of an illness, and no physician is under obligation to make his practice "acceptable" by providing such services. These ways of connecting medical services to personal desires are corruptions of "rights" language under the banner of individualism, which reduces all goods to isolated assertions of rights.

Whatever the rights of patients (and there is surely some minimal list), they do not entail a suspension of the physician's sense of what is good for the patient. To argue thus is merely to state the converse of Aesculapian authority; and that is why no physician, worthy of that name, can provide services "on demand." Such a view assumes either a passive doctor or an adversarial relationship between doctor and patient. It is difficult to appreciate how a therapeutic alliance could blossom in either environment. As Leon Kass has forcefully put it, "the physician's loyalty to his patient must be decidedly qualified by the doctor's loyalty to his art . . . the doctor serves not the patient simply, but, rather the *good* of the patient."[10] In sum, doctors are not free to define the good for patients without their participation, but neither are patients free to impose upon physicians notions of the good which are foreign to the physician's personal values and professional standards.

Any list of "rights" on either side would be, in the final analysis, very short indeed. There are properly no rights for either patients or physicians outside of the commitment by each to a common therapeutic alliance. Rights to life, to treatment, to access, to refuse treatment, to a "natural" death, or even to be treated with dignity are all contingent upon some sense of a common life; none of these is autonomous or automatic. In fact, our "rights" are no more solid than our agreements to uphold them, and they last only so long as together we determine to protect them. Far from being the independent and robust thing they are so often supposed to be, "rights" are actually very delicate and fragile, and not well suited as truncheons to be used against either physicians or patients.

The Meaning of Valid Consent

Among many rights which are currently asserted vis-à-vis medicine, the right to an informed, voluntary, and competent consent is prominent. Why consent enjoys this eminence is an interesting question in itself; but the answer may also display what consent is intended to achieve and accomplish, that is, its telos.

It is of more than casual interest to note that, while the moral traditions of Western medicine contain provisions for a consent mechanism, the influential role of consent as an explicit issue in medical ethics is a relatively recent one. There is only passing reference to the matter, as an extension of physician paternalism, in the *Hippocratic Corpus;*[11] and no mention at all by Maimonides in the twelfth century, or by other pre-nineteenth century medical authorities. Indeed, apart from the Hippocratic concern that "many patients through this cause have taken a turn for the worse," there is no apparent interest among classical medical authorities in a special ethical obligation for physicians with respect to consent, whether regarding experimental or established therapies. Why this is so is uncertain (apart from the enormous limitations of medical interventions until this century), but two reasons can be advanced as viable explanations: the first has to do with human experimentation, and the second with attitudes toward patients which derive from an emphasis on research.

The beginning of human experimentation in the modern period is typically identified with William Harvey's research in human circulation in the early seventeenth century (1628). The great commitments to research as a predominating direction of scientific medicine were not, however, expressed until the mid-twentieth century. Thus, while there has always been curiosity in the clinical setting—and antedating Harvey, to be sure, in the work of Galen and Vesalius and others—it has been in only relatively recent times that clinical investigation has achieved high priority and institutionalization. Concurrently with the rise of research, an intellectual attitude developed in Western culture which had as its principle objective yielding information through systematically designed experiments—a phenomenon we have referred to earlier in discussions of Francis Bacon. This attitude, in turn, provoked conflict and competition with an older principle of primary patient benefit from medical intervention. World War II, and the Nazi medical experiments in particular, exposed the weakness of experimental ethics that were based either solely or largely on scientific advance or social utility; and Nuremberg, although it focused chiefly on experimentation, has become the landmark in the evolution of consent as a prominent issue in the ethics of health care.[12]

Since Nuremberg, it has been generally acknowledged that a patient's (or subject's) valid consent rests upon and consists of three distinct but interrelated elements: information, freedom, and competency. Thus a consent is valid when, and only when, it is secured from a patient (or subject) who is knowledgeable concerning the proposed intervention (or experiment), who agrees voluntarily, and who is compos mentis (or who, in the case of legal or mental incompetency, is represented by a guardian *ad litem*). The pendulum has thereby swung back toward the older principle of primary patient benefit from medical intervention (with the addition of a somewhat newer principle of primary subject protection from scientific investigation); and this, in a word, is the telos of the consent mechanism.

Although many high-technology services are viewed by practitioners as primary care, it is clearly the tendency of medical work in tertiary settings to strengthen the Aesculapian sense of authority and reinforce the idea that only physicians can make sound decisions about patient care. No doubt the high degree of responsibility vested in physicians in these settings contributes to this notion, and this heightened responsibility is accentuated and constantly corroborated by the action-orientation of most tertiary care doctors. Action, even if wrong, clears the air and dispels ambiguity; to fail to act can be viewed as a failure to discharge one's duty; sharing responsibility may be interpreted as *ir*responsibility. The ideals of primary care, in contrast, are meaningless outside of a strong commitment to mutuality; and acceptability of services means that the patient receives or rejects the assistance offered by physicians. Plainly, in the setting of primary care, consent operates as far more than a formal proceeding between patient and physician and is the *ex hypothese* foundation of a thera-peutic relationship.

Perhaps that is why it seems considerably easier, in other medical settings, to treat consent as though it were only a verbal transaction in which the physician attempts to transfer to the patient professional expertise regarding diagnosis, treatment options, and probable out-comes. In any case, it should not be surprising how often this issue is taken up as a matter of saying the right words, dispensing the right information, and thereby subordinating the spirit to the letter of this law. The Aesculapian tradition is understandably skeptical of the value of consent for several resons. The *Hippocratic Corpus,* as we have mentioned, cautions that many patients "have taken a turn for the worse" as a result of being told too much. More recently, it is widely argued (and widely practiced?) that the obligation for valid consent is dispensable when information might become an agent of harm. Every physician who argues this point has his or her own list of compelling memories of occasions on which a valid consent was sought and undesirable results ensued. Occasionally, these are dra-matic scenes in which "curable" patients were so upset when in-formed of their diagnosis that they never returned for treatment and needlessly died. In these situations, we have been told many times, doctors should simply discharge their duty by doing "what is best" for the patient and proceeding with the treatment. The assumption of proceeding thus, of course, is that the physician already has—that is, without patient concurrence—the prerogatives necessary to exercise his private judgment; but that is precisely the assumption which is denied by the argument for the need of consent. (That is also an as-sumption which, undemonstrated in ordinary medical circumstances, makes the physician liable for battery.)

Pellegrino has argued for another understanding of consent: "Con-sent," he says, "grows out of a human interaction between someone who seeks to know what to do and one who advises what should be done."[13] Pellegrino knows that consent means, quite literally, "to feel with" and "to think with" (*cum-sentire*); and he is therefore on solid ground in regarding consent as arising from a commonality *between* patient and physician. Translated into the categories of ethics, a choice of treatment is then "right" when it is medically valid and "good" when it conforms to the patient's values. The contrast, be-tween a traditional model of physician authority which views consent as a possibility to be selectively utilized and the philosophy of primary care which regards consent as a moral imperative for intervention, is thus strikingly stark.

Sometimes it is argued that consent, however desirable, is a practical impossibility, and thereafter follows a litany of problems: patients cannot digest the sophisticated medical understanding which doctors possess; patients have their biases and fears, which frequently render them too anxious to hear what is said much less make an informed choice; some patients simply do not want to be told, but come pliant and dependent to the doctor to be cared for. In these and similar objections, a doctor who would nevertheless seek patients' consents is portrayed as insensitive and legalistic because he forces unwanted news on resisting patients. But to argue this way is to beg the question by confirming the asymmetry of power in the doctor-patient relationship, paying no attention whatever to the harm that is done by concealment, and looking only at the supposed beneficial outcomes. In fact, objections of this sort foreclose on the merits or benefits of consent before it is attempted. Perhaps most important, to argue this way elevates an exception to the status of a universal principle. We do not doubt that some patients prefer not to be informed; but, of course, if *no* patients are informed, the validity of this impression cannot be tested! Moreover, even those who choose not to be informed have exercised, given the opportunity, their prerogative not to know. It therefore appears reasonable that if physicians respect this choice (i.e., not to know), they should correspondingly respect the converse choice (i.e., to be, as fully as possible, informed).

The most persuasive argument by physicians of the Aesculapian school is that consent is redundant and unnecessary. If trust and a therapeutic alliance are present, the consent form is superfluous. On the face of it, the logic is impeccable; in our experience, the "if" is a very large contingency. So the counterargument is forceful as well: if trust and a therapeutic alliance are present between doctor and patient, the consent form will only confirm and make believable to each the intentions of the other. Maurice Merleau-Ponty once remarked that none of us can be certain what we are thinking until we say it; and the explicit consent manifests that dimension of the human condition.

Indeed, we think that the most compelling argument for consent is one which begins with a recognition of the finitude and vulnerability of physician and patient alike. To act in an Aesculapian fashion is to assume a truly godlike burden; the personal requirements of patient care are enormous in any case, but the Aesculapian model makes them Olympian. Only at the cost of suppressing one's own limitations and affective life is it possible, in the long run, to maintain the assumption of total care and total responsibility for patients. We spoke earlier of "detached concern" as a professional norm. Now we can add in this context the common knowledge that physicians, as a group, have higher rates of drug abuse, alcoholism, and suicide than other professional groups—a fact which strongly suggests that, whatever other factors may be contributory, Aesculapian stress is a conspicuous companion of medical practice. Of course we do not mean to suggest that the notion of consent, which we have put forward, is a panacea for this; but we do believe that contemporary American culture cannot support physicians in the Aesculapian paradigm, nor can physicians realistically hope to support themselves and each other if they are truly autonomous possessors of the kind of responsibility which the Aesculapian ideal portrays.

We have argued that the definitions and ideals of primary care fully support the notion of valid consent. It would, in our view, be mistaken, however, to interpret this commitment as an affirmation of individual rights in the liberal tradition. A superficial regard for consent would tend to argue that patient self-determination is important, and that the consent mechanism is simply another instrument by which a patient's rights or individual liberties are enhanced. But to interpret consent in this way is to succumb to a legalistic view of the transaction and reduce the process to a piece of paper which the patient signs. Valid consent, on the other hand, is more appropriately conceived as the *intention* of doctor and patient to be to each other persons, to establish a consensual therapeutic relationship, to form a healing alliance. The consent document, together with all that it reflects, is symbolic of this intention. Knowledge, voluntariness, and competency are the instruments of this intention, apart from which consent becomes trivial and ultimately invalid.

Moral Imagination and Empathetic Identification

The current crisis in physician authority is the crisis of Aesculapian authority attempting to function in an egalitarian and pluralistic ethos. Further complicating that crisis is a patient population which is at best ambiguous and at worst frankly resentful about the sick role. The response of primary care establishes the authority to treat on a new basis of consent, collaboration, and mutuality. This new basis does not depend on some naive recognition of patient parity, or romantic liberal notions of patient autonomy, or mistaken claims of inalienable rights; instead, it depends only upon the recognition, by both doctor and patient, of the special bond and goal of the therapeutic alliance and of the essential humanity which each perceives in the other. Without this recognition, no rule or principle or process or procedure will be of any use; and these can only be hollow forms, void of a center. The novelist-philosopher Iris Murdoch has argued that we can only choose within the world we can see; that is, we can only choose between options which are conceived as possibilities for us.[14] At a deeper level, she argues that moral vision—what we have called "the moral imagination"—lies at the center of our ethics, giving rules and principles their impetus and concepts of the good their backdrop of comprehension. What we argue for here, in the symbolic character of consent and in the deeper reality to which this symbol refers, is precisely that vision of the patient as one with whom one shares a human countenance.

Paul Ramsey has argued forcefully for the notion of the patient as a person, worthy of consent, and of consent as a "canon of loyalty."[15] We agree with the intention and consequence of Ramsey's position, but we are uncertain that the conceptual ideal of "person" can bear the full weight which Ramsey assigns to it. Indeed, to talk of dignity and respect and worth and autonomy in contemporary America will, we think, finally fail because the meaning of this language is hobbled by the classical liberal context in which it came to rhetorical prominence. We prefer to appeal to a more primordial level and rest our case on a sense of community, an intuition of finitude, an awareness of fragility and vulnerability between and among human beings. So Ramsey's system, for all there is to admire in it—and there is much of that—seems to us finally too formal, and ironically *im*personal, to bear up compassionately those persons who are really anxious, in distress, and harmed. In the place of regard and respect, we propose a vision of empathetic identification. The task is not to see *beyond* one's sickness to the dignity of a person, but to see *in* and *through* the sickness the common humanity which physician and patient share alike. Why shouldn't medical ethics be grounded in the instinctual response to help instead of worrying about how to replace that human instinct with a technical concept? As we saw, it was precisely this instinctual identification which motivated the Samaritan; an instinct which finds its justification not in some abstract notion of the good, but from the primitive acknowledgment of mutual vulnerability, and in the depth and scope of our common vision of the human condition.

Despite the best of intentions, consent often fails as both a symbol and a deeper reality. Some of the reasons for this have to do with what we have described as the professional ethos of medicine; some other reasons relate to the liabilities of professional power in a more generic sense. The very conditions which make consent necessary, namely the social status of the physician as authority figure and the asymmetries of power and risk in the physician-patient relationship, also make it difficult to achieve. In the end, our capacity for empathetic identification makes consent possible; our tendency to autonomous power makes consent imperative.

Most discussions of consent tend to take account of power and risk only in relation to whether an *action* is taken. But medical intervention is not limited to physical mediation; physicians are also empowered to intervene in the lives of patients in other, more subtle, ways—by clarifying their illnesses, advising on appropriate courses of action, and even deciding for patients which courses of action are best suited to their diseases. In fact, it is in those shades of difference between clarifying, advising, and deciding that professional values are most likely to preempt the patient's own sense of well-being. Physicians sometimes decide for patients in clarifying an illness; and that action reflects the asymmetry of power. In addition, physicians sometimes do not realize the extent to which clarifying constitutes a mode of deciding; and that failure stems from the asymmetry of risk. The greater the need for help, the less likely it is that the person in need will assert his or her own values and risk losing the attention, care, or ministration of the servicer. Most failures of consent are not failures of effort; still less are they failures of good will or beneficence. Rather they are failures usually based upon an inappropriate sense of authority and an unwillingness or inability to see, more specifically, that not all asymmetries of power can be used for therapeutic ends.

The urgent and enduring question underlying consent is, How is it possible for one person to help another without compounding the problems of the one helped? How can a person be helped without being disgraced, burdened, victimized, oppressed, or ingratiated by receiving help? Perpetuation of the asymmetries of risk and power makes it unlikely that this sort of help can ever be offered. So the answer we are offered is consent, because this is a way of equalizing the relation, closing the power gap, and reducing the risk in the doctor-patient relationship. But this is too simple, and ultimately fails because consent will always be accompanied by ignorance and coercion. Indeed, our experience with physicians in consulting rooms convinces us that the material requirements of valid consent will remain problematic because it is difficult (perhaps, in an absolute sense, impossible) to assess precisely and accurately the extent to which any patient is informed, free, and competent in the consent situation. We have not found any consent situation (not even the possible exception of genuinely elective procedures) which unambiguously satisfies pro forma the full range of interests signified by these elements. Moreover, we do not know of any single rule or principle or protocol which in itself is comprehensive enough to guard all the contingencies, or which by following rigorously would guarantee adequacy.

Consent is therefore, in its deepest sense, an indication that the physician's authority to heal comes ultimately from the patient, and that means also the patient's understanding of his or her illness. Patient consent is the enabling power that is given to physicians, a power which must be confirmed and reconfirmed at every significant juncture in their relationship as a perpetual reminder of how difficult it is to receive help without being victimized by it. To appreciate that the patient's gift comes first, that it is the enfranchising of the physician to treat and the source which turns the physician's considerable power into therapy, is fundamentally important. It reiterates that primary care represents a novel way to practice medicine, and it confirms, especially here, how it is far easier to give than to receive. The point, therefore, is that the patient is the active agent and that the physician, however otherwise authorized, is simply not a physician without the patient's gift. The patient makes the doctor real.

Physicians who recognize that their authority to heal comes from their patients are enabled to exercise power for their patients' well-being without compounding their patients' distress. In this sense, the gratitude of doctor-to-patient and patient-to-doctor is fully mutual: the doctor is made a healer even if he or she fails to cure, and the patient can be grateful for help offered and received in the sure confidence that the physician's skills of intervention have been the gifts of healing. The consent situation therefore offers enormous possibility for covenant between these two. The resulting fiduciary relationship, minimally intended to guard and protect vulnerabilities, may also flourish beyond minimalist duties to confirm the common humanity of both parties. That way of viewing the consent situation is easily forgotten or neglected in the day-to-day routinization of practice (and perhaps especially in the enthusiasm for clinical investigations); but acknowledgment of the consent situation as a covenanting situation will probably go farther than any formal requirement toward respecting both the spirit and the letter of the role of consent.

Each of the cases which follows is based on actual events. The names and other identifying features have been altered, lest we fail in these cases to exemplify one of the chief principles of medical ethics. The cases are all drawn from primary care and are typical of office-based, outpatient care situations.

When cases are presented in a book of this sort, the reader is frequently guided through a list of competing opinions and principles, which are then refined to produce a best solution. We consciously avoid this resolution as being neither sufficient nor true to real life. When we have indicated an outcome, we have done so in recognition that our narrative captures only a fraction of the actual events, and perhaps little of the meaning of those events for the persons whose stories they are.

Still less do we wish, in presenting these cases, to illustrate a favored ethical method. There is, in our opinion, no single best ethical method at present; moreover, to focus the discussion on method distracts from the prime consideration of ethics as moral agency. Methods come into use as helpful tools in the hands of the moral craftsman, not as preconditions or beginning points or conclusions.

Saint-Exupéry said that ". . . a man is but a network of relationships, and these alone matter to him."[1] These cases seek to put on display some of the complexity of that network as it occurs in the primary care physician's practice. As before, our working assumption is that the moral sense of physicians is not formed primarily by the publicly defensive principles they hold, but by the narratives of care in which they recognize themselves as moral agents. The way these problems are perceived and approached will reflect how the moral dimensions of primary care are taken up and used.

So while we call into play some of the basic problem-solving components of ethical reasoning, our purpose in presenting cases is to show how moral strivings draw upon professional senses of self and extend them, through decisions, into therapeutic relationships. It is finally on the meaning of these relationships, rather than on the clarity of principles, that medical ethics rests.

Case 1: For the Patient's Own Good?

A 46-year-old executive has been Dr. M.'s patient for several years. He is a chain smoker, and, despite frequent attempts at helping him to quit, he continues to smoke two packs a day. Finally, Dr. M. elects to send him a letter after a recent physical examination in which he states, "Upon reviewing your chest x-ray with a radiologist, there appears to be early evidence of emphysema." The chest x-ray is actually within normal limits.

The patient stops smoking and in subsequent follow-up visits remains indebted to Dr. M for "changing his life."

All medical cases depict relationships and, as we have argued earlier, it is only in the context of those relationships that moral problems can be properly discerned. William F. May's recent book, *The Physician's Covenant,* provides interesting and helpful images of the physician which presuppose goals for physician-patient relationships and shape subsequent expectations for both parties.[2] May variously depicts physicians as parents, fighters, technicians, and teachers; but all of these are subsumed under the master image of covenantor. We do not know the sort of covenant which, prior to the emphysema letter, obtained between the two parties in our case; and since we do not know, it is difficult to say whether this deception "for the patient's own good" was in keeping with their obligations to each other. Conceivably it could have been; but, on the other hand, perhaps not. In the absence of that important information, we can nevertheless examine whether a physician-patient covenant, in our cultural setting, can appropriately bear the weight of a deception like this one.

Some patients may be genuinely unteachable about their health, in the deep sense of being unable to follow up on advice which they know or ought to know to be in their own best interest. Experience tends to show that smokers are notorious for their resistance to this sort of advice and education. In the case we are considering, we might well argue that the emphysema letter was the last resort, and that it constitutes a justifiable deception. And if this end (stopping smoking) does justify this means (the letter), then invoking the additional authority of radiology to give the lie more impact would be justifiable as well. To use May's categories, here the parent and fighter must prevail since the teacher's role has proved ineffective.

Since Kant we have been accustomed to accept the proposition that the end does not justify the means. That is surely true—even perhaps all of the time. But it is equally true that if anything justifies a means, it is the end which the means serves. That the patient is afterwards grateful could be taken, in that sense, to be vindication of deception as a means because it not only accomplishes the desired end but does so without violating the patient as moral agent.

Yet the fact remains that while the patient's risk of disease is reduced, his present health is technically no different now from what it was last month when he smoked two packs of cigarettes a day. He did not have then, and does not have now, emphysema. He has changed his behavior on information which is, in fact, false. And although he has not been harmed, he has unquestionably been wronged by being lied to. The patient has been used as the track on which the train of the physician's purpose runs. The purpose is a good one, no doubt, and we can assume here the beneficence of motivation. Yet the issue of wronging another remains. The doctor has, in effect, calculated that he was morally justified to wrong the patient in order to help him.

As defense for his actions, Dr. M. could cite the patient's gratitude. One rationale for paternalistic actions is that the person in whose behalf the actions are taken will thank you later. This would require, however, that Dr. M. disclose the deception at some later point. If thereafter the patient still thanks Dr. M., and approves of being deceived for this purpose, then there may be genuine validation. The thanks Dr. M. accrues now, though it may be deeply felt, is impotent to justify the deception because it is a gratitude created *by* the deception.

It could be argued that Dr. M. had a tacit consent to deceive. The patient does want to stop smoking, or at least that is implied by the suggestion of "frequent attempts." A contract to help a patient stop smoking could have anticipated wielding the power of labeling and diagnosis in keeping the contract. Yet whether such a contract, leaving implicit the morality of the means used to keep it, can itself be justified is questionable. Covenants which might include in them a contract to lie, when other means fail, may so stretch our sense of covenantal fidelity as to license almost anything.

One additional impact of such a decision should not go unnoticed, and that is the impact upon the physician himself. The assumption of authority exhibited in the care of this patient has implications for Dr. M.'s sense of his role and authority for other patients. It is not that the happy ending portrayed here (so far) may not be replicated in other cases. It is rather that lack of respect for patient self-determination in one area of care or with one patient can lead to similar moral agency in other areas of care, and with other patients. The fact that it "worked" may make it all the more tempting. Even were such moral agency justified, this case is exceptional and should not become a precedent for "managing" other "noncompliant" patients. For just to couch the case in this language is to beg the question and forego the tension inherent in this situation as a genuine ethical problem.

Finally, we should ask whether other options were fully considered. Hypnosis and other behavior modification programs do work for some, and are morally preferable because of their voluntariness and lack of deceit. Medical care produces relationships of all sorts, with varying degrees of trust, authority, needs, power balances and imbalances, and each has actions internally consistent to its well-being and its continuation as a therapeutic alliance. Whether Dr. M.'s action or any similar action is justifiable will finally depend upon the covenant which is established. It would be, however, a rare instance to find a physician-patient relationship which could bear the weight of a deception as major as this one.

Case 2: Divided Loyalties in Family Practice?

Mr. and Mrs. C. were patients in Dr. K.'s family practice. In the course of annual physical examination, customary blood serology studies revealed that Mrs. C. was positive for gonorrhea. Mr. C.'s serology was negative. Dr. K. was troubled about how to manage this situation: Mrs. C. had not intended to reveal an extramarital affair to Dr. K., and would not have done so voluntarily and verbally; Mr. C. was also Dr. K.'s patient and should be protected from the infection. Dr. K. believed that he could not, however, violate the confidential relationship between himself and Mrs. C. by informing Mr. C. Dr. K. considered several alternatives, among which were drugs resistant to the gonococcus bacterium for Mr. C. and fabricating reasons why Mr. and Mrs. C. should abstain from sexual intercourse during the infectious period.

If it is true that good answer-getting is a function of good question-asking, this case offers a particularly fertile illustration of that maxim. The typical tendency, in our experience, in discussion of this case is to offer objections to the facticity of the case ("But doing a blood serology is not customary in a routine annual physical"); and thereafter to propose *a* principle ("Patient confidentiality is a sacred trust and cannot be violated"—sometimes with the codicil, "except under the most extenuating circumstances") which is supposed to depress other troublesome aspects, and settle the matter cleanly.

When discussion of this case proceeds along these lines, a long list of competing principles is quickly developed ("Dr. K.'s obligation is to his primary patient" or "Dr. K.'s first duty is to do no harm"), in consequence of which it appears that only an arbitrary selection of one of these competing notions can resolve the matter— but at the obvious expense of leaving other aspects unattended because the rule doesn't fit or address them. What actually occurred in this case may illustrate better than subsequent discussions of it how physicians can enter situations like this as full moral agents and employ the tools of ethics to describe moral experience and move toward acceptable resolutions.

Dr. K. suspected, soon after receiving the blood serologies for both Mr. and Mrs. C., that he had somewhat inadvertently stumbled upon a bit of information which Mrs. C. had not intended to reveal to him. That suspicion was confirmed by Mrs. C.'s obvious embarrassment and discomfort when he reported, as he had always done before, the findings of the annual physical examination to her. She reluctantly acknowledged that she had indeed engaged in extramarital sexual intercourse, and she went on to say several important things about that "indiscretion," as she called it: that this was the first and only time, that she had just allowed herself to be overcome by curiosity for this "forbidden excursion," that she deeply loved her husband and children, and that she did not want this—the only thing of its sort in seventeen years of marriage—to destroy the close and cherished relationships between herself and her husband and family.

"What to do?" was a question attended by some urgency for both Dr. K. and Mrs. C. Therapy for the infection needed to be begun immediately; beyond that, however, Mr. C., out of town on business today, was returning tomorrow and had a follow-up appointment with Dr. K. in the late afternoon. After considering several alternatives with Mrs. C., Dr. K. proposed two courses of action: that they begin drug therapy for Mrs. C. and that together they talk with a priest. Mrs. C. agreed to both proposals.

As it turned out, Dr. K.'s insight into the moral significance of Mrs. C.'s problem—that her situation involved her most cherished relationships and the values attendant to them—was critical for its resolution. After having been acquainted with the situation, the priest questioned Mrs. C. about her understanding of her marriage and her intentions toward her husband. When it was clear that Mrs. C. very much wanted to preserve her marriage, and that she understood and intended herself to be wife and mother in her family, the priest suggested that the parties concerned—Dr. K., Mrs. C., Mr. C., and himself—discuss the matter openly at the earliest opportunity. That, in fact, happened the following afternoon; and without detailing the conversation (or its choreography), the situation was satisfactorily resolved. Concretely that meant that Mr. and Mrs. C. were reconciled and renewed their marriage vows, and that Dr. K. proceeded to treat both his patients for the bacterial infection.

No one associated with this case supposes that certain irreducible risks were not the accompaniment of every decision along the way; or that things might have turned out quite differently than they did. So while there was general satisfaction, both about what happened and why it happened, there was also the sober recognition that ethically charged situations are not soluble by the simple application of rules and principles. Engagement of persons as moral agents, who have sensibilities about who they are and what they really cherish when the chips are down, was at stake in this case. And honesty (whether between the physician and patient or between a wife and husband), or fairness (in regard to competing patient claims, or marital harmony), or any other principle or rule was thereby employed *instrumentally;* that is, the agents in this case used the tools of ethical inquiry and advocacy to accomplish a *telos,* an end or goal which together they shared.

Alasdair MacIntyre has convincingly argued that we do not have a rational method for resolving moral dispute in this society because we do not share a common tradition and commonly held values.[3] This case is illustrative of the importance of shared traditions and commonly held notions about what is worthwhile. With that consensus, these moral agents could agree upon the goal they all sought (in this case, actually two goals related and complementary: physical and marital health); and the means they chose for resolution, while not without some evident risk, nevertheless offered larger promise of achieving their mutual goal than would have been the case had they not shared the same *telos*.

This case also illustrates that there are boundaries—not always easily or simply defined—to professional competence; and that sometimes physicians (as well as other professionals) can and should usefully employ others who stand in a different relationship and whose skills lie elsewhere than in medicine for accurate identification of pathologies and effective therapeutic intervention. Finally, in this case, the presence of the gonococcus bacterium was surely real enough and a sufficient warrant for medical therapy; but in a larger personal sense, the bacterium was symptomatic of another kind of pathology—that of a marriage on the edge of serious problems. "Family practice" in particular, and "primary care" in general, are appropriately alert to this larger perspective because they are committed to a concept of health which embraces the whole person.

Case 3: Continuing Placebos for Long-Range Benefits?

Mrs. Jones gives a history suggestive of a mild depression, but otherwise appears to be enjoying good health. There are no unusual findings on the physical examination. "But doctor," she says, "why do I have to feel so bad then? Before I moved here, Dr. X. used to give me a shot every month that made me feel a lot better. It was a B-12 shot." Mrs. Jones requests that you continue to give her the shots, as Dr. X. did.

You believe that the drug has no therapeutic value for Mrs. Jones except, perhaps, its placebo effect. However, the patient would undoubtedly leave your office happy and feeling better if you gave her the shot. She would probably return regularly, opening the possibility of long-term therapy.

Patients' perceptions of the ability of medicine to cure is a powerful factor in their overall care. Without widespread belief in the efficacy of scientific medicine, many medications would, in fact, not be as effective. The placebo effect accounts for a significant portion of the potency of pharmacologically active drugs, and for all the healing power of inert medications, such as sugar pills and B-12 shots.[4] But sometimes this belief is misplaced or exaggerated, schooling dependency in patients and perhaps even abusive habits with regard to medication.

The potential for excessive reliance on medicine is especially acute as technology adds more machines and medications, of both proven and dubious benefit, to the physician's armamentarium. Given this general cultural scenario, should Mrs. Jones get her B-12 shots, or not?

In one sense Mrs. Jones is committing a cardinal sin—prescribing for herself. Though she could buy B-12 over the counter, giving herself injections would be more difficult, and in any case, not getting it from the doctor would destroy a good deal of the placebo value. She is, moreover, attempting to dictate her own treatment, in a deeper way. Her remarks about Dr. X. are meant as something of a challenge: "Are you as concerned for me as he was?" She means to instruct her new physician that concern is measured in prescription pads, injections, or other magic in the physician's black bag. Physicians, like all professionals, usually resent being told their business or manipulated into a course of action they would not otherwise choose. Mrs. Jones' plea indicates that the doctor holds the key to her wellbeing. Her complaint that she feels bad *unnecessarily* is intended to evoke the compassion which unlocks the cabinet with the hypodermics. How to deal with manipulative patients of all sorts is a continuing challenge. Assertions of professional prerogative—"I'm the doctor here"—do little except bluntly affirm what the patient's ploy already acknowledges—that the doctor holds most of the power, and that the patient must make an acceptable presentation of suffering to ensure that her needs are met.

Such a patient as Mrs. Jones could be swayed in her views about B-12, but these efforts will almost surely fail, at least initially. The key to long-term care, and the building of a more adequate basis of care and education, lies in providing this woman what she wants. Otherwise one can almost guarantee a sequence of doctor-shopping culminating in a relationship with a physician who caters to, or at least doesn't mind meeting, her perceived needs.

Mrs. Jones seems to have little faith in the doctor now; rather her faith is in the medication, and the doctor is but the means to obtain it. Whether she can be converted to another allegiance—and even if she can, whether she should be—are the central questions. Given the relative harmlessness of monthly B-12 injections (and the probability that she will get them somewhere anyway) agreeing initially to this "therapy" could well be a low-risk way of establishing a long-term contract.

Underlying the need for B-12, however, is a personal need, a gap or an imbalance in Mrs. Jones' life. Time is required to find out what that is, and to assess whether there are better ways for her to cope with her problems. While the injections may be relatively innocuous now, the pattern of dependency upon medication to rectify one's well-being and meet the routine problems of living is a dangerous one. Physicians are tempted to foster such dependence rather than probe beneath it. Exercising what Michael Balint calls "apostolic function,"[5] and converting Mrs. Jones to healthier responses to stress or loss, will require time. Convincing her to be less dependent on medicine may take even longer, or be impossible. The shots, if contracted for along with other therapy, seem like a small token to offer until some other symbols can be substituted or the needs alleviated. Careful review at regular intervals would be a necessity for a pact of this sort, as would a full disclosure of the physician's reservations about her current enthusiasm for the B-12. Approaching her depression is the ultimate goal, and this will need to be done even if it scares her away to a more compliant doctor.

Additional issues could be raised about whether and how much to charge Mrs. Jones for something which is essentially a placebo. If one charges for its effectiveness or value to the patient, the price would be hefty: while not charging her at all, or only a small fee, would be more in keeping with the medical understanding of its value. This is a significant decision because placebos, in order to work, must be obtained at some cost, however modest. Psychiatrists have known for some time that talk is truly cheap if not charged for, and that paying the bill is a part of getting well. Professional courtesy is usually not operative in psychiatry for just this reason—that it vitiates the therapy!

Clarifying intentions and motives, on the part of both the physician and the patient, may be more important here than in other situations. A critical long-range test may be whether the physician retains Mrs. Jones in his practice if his efforts to probe her deeper problems fail. Excusing or dismissing her, unless it is to more expert help, would not give due regard to the need for loyalty, especially to those labeled neurotics or "crocks." These sorts of cases are a potent reminder that covenants to help, like marriages, frequently lead to places we did not foresee or anticipate; and yet we are responsible to and for them all the same.

Case 4: Adolescent Confidentiality?

Michael is a 12-year-old 7th grader who comes in for a sports physical. In the course of the history he admits to smoking pot. He indicates that he and a friend routinely share a joint on the way to school and pop a variety of pills once in a while. He is doing poorly in school, and does not seem alarmed by either his school performance or his drug use. His mother gives no indication of knowing about her son's drug use.

Pediatricians, especially those who treat adolescents, occasionally find themselves in situations of divided loyalty or ambiguous obligations. Case 4 presents the problem of whether to tell the mother about her son's drug use. Arguments can be made on both sides of the case.

The case for telling will likely seem more compelling to the adult reader, since we tend naturally to empathize with the parent. Moreover, the reasons for sharing this information with the mother are strong ones. First, parents are legally responsible for their minor children, and failure to tell the parents compromises their ability to act responsibly on the child's behalf. A possible consequence of failing to inform the mother is that the physician may risk a lawsuit.

A second and more substantial reason is that therapy may depend upon the mother's help. Relationships between parents and their children vary enormously; but for many patients like Michael, exclusion of the parents would handicap the physician's ability to follow through with care, even with such mundane matters as scheduling and getting Michael to a next appointment. Twelve-year-olds have obviously limited capacities to initiate and maintain continuity in treatment.

The correlation between drug use and poor school performance should not go unnoticed. If the mother already suspects the use of drugs, she would be unlikely to believe anything but a confirmation of that as fact, should she ask the physician.

From a purely fiscal standpoint it could be argued that the mother is entitled to the information because she pays the bill. Though not an argument which stands alone, the financial contract is with the parent to care for the child. Beyond any legal obligations to provide for children, however, there are important moral requirements which derive from the parent-child bond. The decision to have children is taken, in this society, to be sufficient warrant for requiring the parent to assume certain responsibilities to and for the child. Making contracts and paying bills on behalf of a child are among the evidences of the deeper relationship which binds the parent and child to each other. To argue that the mother is entitled to this information because she pays the bill is not therefore incorrect, but it is inadequate by itself to account for the relationships or moral agency out of which this obligation to pay and its corresponding entitlement to know derive.

Although difficult to interpret, Michael's admission to drug use is possibly a signal that he wants his parents to know, hasn't found a way to tell them, and assumes that the doctor will inform them for him. The doctor can make the news safe, perhaps by medicalizing it and softening the moral force of parental judgment and disapproval.

The case for not telling Michael's mother has its appeal also. Confidentiality is a medical-moral maxim as old as Hippocrates, and it is universally recognized. The assumption of confidentiality is essential to most patients and breaches of this undertanding are reason, at a minimum, to change doctors. The reasons for not keeping a confidence must be compelling and the burden of proof is on those who wish to justify the exception, not on those who favor upholding the norm.

Besides the respect of the individual patient which undergirds confidentiality, there is a strong consequentialist argument for doctors keeping secrets. Loss of faith in doctors' ability or willingness to guard information makes us less likely to seek help when we need it, or to tell the full story when we do. For example, it is well known that the so-called "squeal law," requiring doctors to inform parents when their minor children seek contraceptive advice, turned some teenagers away and resulted in unwanted pregnancies. Without help, patients suffer; with help based on partial information, both patient and doctor are likely to suffer or commit needless mistakes in diagnosis or therapy. Accomplished clinicians repeatedly say that the patient history is three-fourths of the diagnosis in ambulatory care. Partial histories compromise both doctor and patient. Hence, patient assumptions of confidentiality are indispensable.

Telling the mother could jeopardize the physician's ability to do anything at all, or worse, drive Michael away from medical advice indefinitely. An assurance of confidentiality could seal the sort of covenant Michael needs with an adult.

Though the financial contract is between the physician and the mother, the therapeutic covenant must be between the physician and Michael. The parents can be an effective part of this only to the extent that Michael wishes. That is another evidence of the moral dimensions of the parent-child bond.

One possible resolution is to bring Michael into the decision about whether to inform his mother. This could be done in a variety of ways: (1) actually leaving the decision altogether up to him; (2) advising him that it is important and must be done unless he has compelling reasons that his mother should not know; (3) telling him that his mother must know and leaving it to Michael as to when, how, and who informs her. All these options respect his autonomy, to varying degrees.

On the whole we tend toward disclosing this information to the mother; or if that is truly impossible (e.g., Michael is at risk for physical abuse), a school counselor, minister, or someone in whom Michael has confidence. The point is that Michael needs an advocate outside the physician's office and if not the parents, then someone else must be found.

A final issue remains, and that is the physician's responsibility to the larger school and community. Drug traffic constitutes a bona fide health hazard to the larger society. Locating the sources and alerting principals, school boards, law enforcement officials, and public health workers constitutes the fulfillment of larger covenants between physicians and society to strive for a public good beyond individual patient care.

Case 5: Work Release for a Troubled Marriage?

A 25-year-old manual laborer visits your office for the first time. His presenting problem is a badly bruised and abraded left hand, with a small hematoma on the back of the hand. No fractures are evident from x-ray studies, and you reassure him and offer him a five-day work release. Without hesitation the patient says he needs two weeks off. When you ask, "Why?" he replies that his wife has run away to Arizona. He needs two weeks off to find her and bring her home. He confesses that he had beaten his own hand with a brick in order to gain access to a physician and obtain a medical leave.

The "insanity plea" has received increasingly voluble criticism over recent years; and there are strong pressures from several quarters, including medicine, for revision of both medical and legal assessment of accountability in this regard. The case of this laborer's self-mutilation does not qualify under the legal provisions for diminished responsibility, but it does contain elements which raise that issue as the physician considers an appropriate response.

Through the early decades of this century, the capacity of physicians to intervene in the presence of illness or injury was, certainly when compared with current capabilities, very limited indeed. That was so in large part because the extraordinary achievements in biomedical technology and the remarkable advances in drug and other therapies, which we tend nowadays to take so much for granted, had not yet occurred. But a limited capacity to intervene was also the case because of two additional factors: The emergence of psychiatry as a bona fide medical speciality was still somewhat aborning; and the concept of omnibus medicine, from which virtually no aspect of human somatic and psychic well-being was to be exempt, awaited those dramatic technologies and therapies which were gathering momentum at about midcentury.

These factors help us to understand that while medicine depends upon scientific and technical apparatus, it is also supported by social sanctions which authorize the extent of intervention. So while scientific and technical achievements are acknowledged, it is also important to appreciate developments in other spheres as contributory to the ways we presently set both expectations and limitations. In this context, the single example of the Durham Rule is instructive: That rule, formulated in 1954, stated that a person is not criminally responsible if unlawful behavior is the product of mental disease or mental defect. The bearing of that rule on the "insanity plea" is doubtless obvious; but we mention it here to illustrate those nonscientific and nontechnical factors which currently influence, and impinge upon, medical practice. The impact of the Durham Rule is certain, even if one can't recall its name; and because of it, the physician in this case can entertain a number of questions and alternative courses not immediately signified by physical diagnosis. To put it plainly, the physician in this case is not bound by either medical or legal or social conventions to be merely a technician; in this case he or she is also confronted with the practice of medicine as an art.

Treatment of the injury to the back of the hand, barring unexpected complications, is relatively straightforward. It is the further request for additional time off from work, together with the etiology of the injury itself, which appropriately gives the physician pause. Is this injury the product of an act both conscious and unconscious? Is the patient punishing himself for some reason? Because his wife has run away? Because he has in some way provoked her leaving? Because he beat her, perhaps out of the same kind of frustration which prompted him to injure himself? Does he want just to extricate himself so that he can hunt for his wife? Will he be successful in finding her? Will it be a good thing if he does find her? Would granting his request constitute a dishonest and fraudulent abuse of the provisions for medically indicated work release? Can rules always satisfactorily take account of the human dimensions of problems? Should you insist upon a more thorough evaluation of this patient, either by yourself or a psychiatrist or psychologist, before granting or denying his request? How much do you need to know about *why* he injured himself, and *why* his wife ran away to Arizona, before you can make an intelligent and appropriate decision?

We are told by our friends who are engaged in primary care practices that this series of questions, together with some others which space doesn't permit, would probably be asked by a conscientious physician. What is most interesting about these questions is that they probe behind the *what* to the *why;* that is, they focus on what it means to be a moral agent, on where loyalties and convictions about what is right and wrong, helpful and harmful, proper and improper, appropriate and inappropriate belong in consideration of concrete courses of action.

We think that this case nicely demonstrates how it is that sometimes more information and knowledge is needed and wanted before some decisions can be made. Even if a five-day work release is routinely given for an injury of this sort, that decision is not neat and clean in view of the request for more time off and the ostensible reasons which the laborer gives. Had the conversation ended with the offer (and acceptance) of a five-day work release, the physician would be relieved of further responsibility (barring, of course, unexpected complications with the hematoma). But the additional information from the laborer introduces a disclosure to the physician-patient relationship which is not accessible by physical examination, x-ray, diagnosis, and ordinary care.

At times medical ethics introduces a tragic dimension. Medicine is unavoidably engaged by problems which sometimes seem to be beyond the powers of even our best efforts to resolve. There are elements of the tragic dimension in this case, not because some of the issues which confront us here represent a failure of reason but because these issues stretch beyond where reason can go. There is no certain way, for example, for us to know precisely what "the good" or "the appropriate" means in a situation like this; and we cannot predict with much precision what the consequences of a decision (to grant a five-day work release, or a two-week work release, or delay either until fuller evaluation, or whatever) might be for all concerned. So this case is tragic because the good we would do, we may not be able to do—partly because we lack knowledge, but chiefly because we lack precise moral foresight. And the consequence of that recognition is that the physician, in ways not dissimilar to the laborer and his estranged wife, will be unable to deal with these matters as might be done with an algebraic equation; instead, both he and they will be obliged just to live through, or live out, this situation. That, as we suggested earlier, need not be interpreted negatively or as defeating; it is simply acknowledgment of an essential part of the human condition, and surely as full of promise as of peril.

5 ◇ Primary Care and Social Justice

Every profession is legitimated by the good faith it keeps with the people it serves. That is why, in our reflections on ethics and primary care, we have directed principal attention toward the character of professionals (in this case, physicians) who not only claim, but are also justified by, public trust. That is also how the principles of virtue within medicine—the larger ratio of benefit over harm through intervention, the placement of patient well-being above the physician's personal or material gain, and the like—are among the essential ways in which medicine, as a profession, secures and maintains its viability within a just and humane society.

This covenant of good faith with those served is, however, only part of the professional charge. Together with the principles of virtue are all of those ways in which the principles are acted out in the practice of virtue. So an equally important aspect of professional legitimation has to do with who is served and how that service is provided: with whom is this covenant of good faith made, and how is it actually expressed in professional practice? This is a question of justice.

In raising the question of justice we are making a major shift in emphasis from the individual to the social level. It is not an easy shift, and it requires self-conscious effort. It means placing oneself outside the ordinary boundaries of relationships with particular patients and colleagues in order to ask about one's position in the larger social order. In our experience, this is typically not done effortlessly, perhaps especially for physicians, because the medical profession has tended to confine its ethical deliberations to concerns about individual behavior in one-to-one relationships. Nor is it made less difficult by a long tradition of thinking about ethics which has ignored questions of justice.

Ethics and Individual Rights

Those of us in American culture experience this predicament because we have been nourished, for the most part, in traditions of bootstrap individualism and independence. Philip Slater has given classic expression to this powerful motif in our sensibilities:

Once upon a time there was a man who sought escape from the prattle of his neighbors and went to live alone in a hut he had found in the forest. At first he was content, but a bitter winter led him to cut down the trees around his hut for firewood. The next summer he was hot and uncomfortable because his hut had no shade, and he complained bitterly of the harshness of the elements.

He made a little garden and kept some chickens, but the rabbits were attracted by the food in the garden and ate much of it. The man went into the forest and trapped a fox, which he tamed and taught to catch rabbits. But the fox ate up the man's chickens as well. The man shot the fox and cursed the perfidy of the creatures of the wild.

The man always threw his refuse on the floor of the hut and soon it swarmed with vermin. He then built an ingenious system of hooks and pulleys so that everything in the hut could be suspended from the ceiling. But the strain was too much for the flimsy hut and it soon collapsed. The man grumbled about the inferior construction of the hut and built himself a new one.

One day he boasted to a relative in his old village about the peaceful beauty and plentiful game surrounding his forest home. The relative was impressed and reported back to his neighbors, who began to use the area for picnics and hunting excursions. The man was upset by this and cursed the intrusiveness of human beings. He began posting signs, setting traps, and shooting at those who came near his dwelling. In revenge groups of boys would come at night from time to time to frighten him and steal things. The man took to sleeping every night in a chair by the window with a loaded shotgun across his knees. One night he turned in his sleep and shot off his foot. The villagers were saddened by this misfortune and thereafter stayed away from his part of the forest. The man became lonely and cursed the unfriendliness and indifference of his former neighbors. And all these troubles the man saw as coming from outside himself, for which reason, and because of his technical skills, the villagers called him the American.[1]

Slater's parable of the American finds its paradigmatic ethical expression in terms of *rights*. In recent decades, the agenda for social change has been couched increasingly in terms of rights of many and varied sorts. Civil rights, women's rights, and gay rights have received the most attention; but a growing chorus has begun to chant the litany of patients' rights—the rights of ill children, of hospital patients, of those who refuse treatment, and of those who are dying— as well as the umbrella right, the right to health care. Ironically, amid all these assertions of rights, the 1980 AMA "Principles" affirmed a number of rights for physicians. In our time, and to a greater extent than ever before, rights talk has become a rite. Can it also be cogently argued that the rights talk with which we are so familiar is well-founded and useful in human and social intercourse?

The development of rights-language is a logical extension of the ideas of our philosophical forebears John Locke and Thomas Jefferson. Locke, together with the American founding fathers, adhered to a notion of "natural rights" and listed those rights that all persons could rationally demand.[2] Among these are "life," "liberty," and "property." Rights, in this sense, are not merely things we claim, but things we validly insist upon by virtue of our human (or other special) status. Because modern Western culture is highly pluralistic and individualistic, it seems to many persons altogether appropriate that the primary rights are those intended to remove barriers to, or infringements upon, individual freedoms.

What we have tended to ignore is that, for this nation, our founders envisioned a society which would offer *both* liberty *and* justice for all. There is thus a tension created between these two grand concepts in our social and political rhetoric, whereby "liberty" and "justice" qualify and constrain each other, and neither is appropriately defined for our situation without reference to the other. That is why a dictionary definition of liberty (the condition of being not subject to restriction or control; the right to act in a manner of one's own choosing) won't wash; that is also why a pedestrian notion of justice as "giving each his due" is ingenuous. Our national history is illustrative of the difficulties inherent in achieving equilibrium between liberty and justice, as sometimes we have emphasized one and sometimes the other. How to attain a stable balance seems still to be somewhat problematic.

Ronald Dworkin captures the tone of contemporary rhetoric in calling rights "political trumps held by individuals."[3] In the current climate, rights are often used as truncheons to club one's opponent. In our time and circumstance, rights have taken on an absolutist temper, and become the weapons of moral debate (or castigation) wielded by individuals as claims against others. From an original position which affirmed rights as freedom-from interference, we have moved steadily toward a rights-language which affirms entitlement to a freedom-for an expanded range of social and economic goods.

Recourse to an individualized and absolutist notion of rights is no stranger to medical care; indeed, this tactic is frequently used as a conversation-stopper in ethical disputes. Patients sometimes claim an absolute right to care, or to the best treatment available; conversely, physicians claim absolutely the right to serve whom they choose as a basic professional prerogative. When absolute rights clash absolutely, ethics is dead in the water.

We maintain that the idea of rights as "trumps held by individuals" is only one dimension of the moral sense of rights. When taken by itself, such a view distorts and cripples other key notions of moral life. Considerations of responsibility and accountability, for example, and more generally the role and relationships of persons in larger communal orders of living, raise issues of justice which provide a more comprehensive and satisfactory moral perception of rights.

It is easy to see why rights-language has become the ethical idiom of choice in America. It has a great legacy in our political philosophy and professional rhetoric. But it is also easy to see how rights-language, in contemporary formulations, does not serve us well. When mixed with the contemporary seasoning of individualism and moral absolutism, the legacy and its rhetoric become malformed by misproportion. What is missing is recognition that rights are secured to individuals by the community. This acknowledgment not only leads to a different understanding of rights, but to a different understanding of persons as holders of rights. In this altered context, rights lose some of their pristine absoluteness and thereby take an appropriate place in moral discourse. In what follows, we will argue for a notion of rights which embraces both individual liberties and some lively sense of social interdependence.

For H. L. A. Hart, a right is something to be taken into account, not an obligation or duty either to undertake or to refrain from a specific action.[4] Joel Feinberg says that rights are the *grounds* of obligations.[5] And while he thinks that rights generally imply correlative duties, it would be simplistic to think that the mere assertion of a right somehow settles issues like the distribution of scarce medical resources, or physician-patient confidentiality in family practice. Ascribing rights may be only a first step; a second and necessary step is deciding what the ascription of rights to certain persons amounts to, and what actions (if any) can licitly follow.

Rights are logically anterior to specific claims, and are not themselves claims on others. In other words, rights—such as a right to health care, or a right to professional autonomy—form the foundation for moral argument, but are never conclusive until their range of application(s) is specified and established. The task imposed by rights-language thus requires a more careful delineation of the scope and range of application(s) of a right, as that right is brought into play in particular instances. It is precisely this sort of work, essential to make practical sense of rights, which is preempted by the absolutist doctrine of rights.

Rights, in the moral sense, clearly are not "trump cards" which individuals may use to exercise tyranny over a moral dispute. In actual practice, the use of rights as "trump cards" by adversaries frequently results in stalemate, since neither person is willing (or for that matter, knows how) to yield anything to the other. Failure to recognize that rights are secured to persons by the community leads invariably to individual assertion of private privilege, arrogance, and independence; with the result that the parties to a dispute are unable rationally to resolve their differences. In such a case, this inability is constant and pervasive, and conflict gets settled accordingly by power: if one party is more powerful than another, he simply tyrannizes his opponent by installing and enforcing his right; if both parties are approximately equal in power, and each thereby powerless to overcome the other, the issue stands still in the water while they agree to disagree. Therefore, whether by tyranny or stalemate, this way of dealing with moral disputes over alleged rights leaves us in the uncomfortable and untenable position of affirming that "might makes right."

Instead of viewing rights as "trump cards" or truncheons, and for all the sovereignty which rights *might* claim in adjudicating controversy, rights are rather more like the foundations of a moral superstructure to which persons in a moral dispute may appeal and on which specific moral actions rely for their justification. To treat rights as absolute possessions, which individuals may exercise at their private discretion, is both to abuse the concept of rights and to misunderstand the role and status of rights in moral argument. Ascriptions of rights are a different kind of moral discourse from judgments about what one ought to do.

To say that rights are not absolutes is not to say that rights are relative and slack, or that they can be compromised or altered or upheld only when convenient. To assert the nonabsolutist character of rights is not to embrace relativism; indeed, the allegation of relativism simply misses the point. Similarly, we do not reject individualism out-of-hand; but we do argue that the private and possessive connotations of contemporary autonomous individualism distort the use of rights-language in moral disputes.

The purpose of ascriptions of rights in moral argument is to delineate some aspects of what it means to be distinctively human. When rights are appealed to, it is those distinctively human aspects of moral alternatives which are highlighted; or, to put it differently, it is the shape of our general self-understanding which is evoked. Most rights, for example, are thought to apply to persons irrespective of social class, economic condition, race, religion, or other contingent circumstance. And what we call natural rights, or human rights, are thought to be anterior to social contracts and professional role obligations. Indeed, in Western democracies, professions are supposed to derive their just powers from their fidelity to the natural rights of those whom the professions serve.

In contrast to the conventional ideology of rights as individualized absolutes, we contend that rights are social and relational. The exercise of personal rights and social interdependence are inseparable aspects of human life; and that is why individual freedom is a social reality. What is needed, therefore, is a notion of rights which values individual prerogatives within a lively sense of social order. Rights cannot be understood outside their social ethos—and this is a theme to which we will return later.

Meanwhile, it is important to recognize that the result of our heritage of individual rights is neglect of significant issues of justice. Because we have been encouraged to view the social order as an aggregate of individuals, and not as a social unity, ethics has been collapsed into individual cases of right or wrong; and one need look no further than the books and articles on medical ethics which were produced in the last decade for proof of this approach. We lack a strong tradition of social ethics because we do not recognize ourselves as belong-ing, in any definitive and primordial sense, to a just society. The En-lightenment paradigm of free and rational men, coming together to form a political order out of convenience and for mutual gain, is so deeply written on our national character that themes of interdepen-dence and mutuality lie dormant. Like the American in Slater's para-ble, we tend to think of our actions as atomic, isolated, and void of social meaning.

In the absence of such a communal and connected sense, obliga-tions to the poor or disenfranchised appear as only individual duties which are sponsored by largesse, philanthropy, or noblesse oblige. They do not, and logically cannot, appear as concerns of social justice because justice, in a social order which is only or even chiefly an ag-gregate of individuals, is solely a function of individual virtues and prerogatives. The traditions of medical ethics, both past and present, are characteristically silent on issues of justice for precisely this rea-son. The 1980 "Principles" of the AMA urge the physician to con-tribute to his community, but as a private citizen; they also advocate appropriate patient care, but simultaneously guarantee the physician freedom in choosing whom to serve. There is no hint that physicians, or the medical profession as a whole, might have obligations to influ-ence the distribution of medical resources to serve the underserved. On the contrary, those portions of the "Principles" which venture toward recognition of interdependency and mutuality forcefully re-iterate the individual practitioner's sovereignty over how he shall use his professional skills.

Similar traits, we might add, appear in other professional codes as well; and were we addressing professional ethics and their sensibili-ties for social justice in a more general way, we could cite compara-ble examples from law, business, engineering, and the like. So while we are addressing doctors in this book, we do not mean to imply that physicians are unique among American professionals in their studied avoidance of social justice questions. As we have indicated, physicians have only reflected the predominant American sensibility in these matters; and, to the extent that medical codes and practices have avoided issues of justice, so have we all.

The Nature of Justice

To inquire about justice is a sophisticated task. It means that we must bracket or suspend our obsession with individual rights in order to look at the social order. To ask about justice is, by definition, to place ourselves in a communal setting.

Concern with individual moral choices leads us to ask: What actions are good? What should a physician do? Concern with the character of virtue of physicians leads us to ask: What makes for good persons? How is medical sensibility rightly formed? How is professional imagination properly animated and enlivened? Concern for the larger community leads us to ask: What constitutes the good society? and, How may physicians collectively serve the common good?

In previous chapters we have endeavored to show how decisions can be understood only within the framework of character, virtues, and the moral imagination. "What should I do?" is inexorably bound up with "Who am I (as a physician)?" In this chapter the question "Who am I as a physician?" is extended to mean, "Who are physicians in this society?" Defining the good in relation to life in the larger community completes ethics and prevents it from becoming parochial. It is this third set of questions which deals with justice.

Justice can be contemplated in a variety of ways. In its simplest sense, it means treating similar cases in a similar fashion. We use the term "unjust" in a general sense to mean "unfair," that is, to refer to actions or policies that are discriminatory. When equals receive unequal treatment, we say that the inequality is arbitrary and, hence, unjust. Reparative or restorative justice seeks to correct for past harms and to restore a proper balance to the ill-served segments of society. "Affirmative Action" programs in recruitment and hiring are obvious examples of reparative justice. The major concern of medicine today is *distributive justice;* that is, the fair distribution of medical goods and service. Such a concern, of course, presumes a condition of scarcity. Distributive justice would not be a problem if there were enough goods and services for everyone; if there were no scarcity, there would be no competing claims.

But what is just; and how is justice to be measured? In distributing scarce medical goods and services, on what basis shall we decide? A purely egalitarian system would embody the letter of the law in justice, but not its spirit, and provide everybody with an equal measure of everything. "Good health" is among the things most unevenly distributed in our society, perhaps because so many personal and social and biological variables affect the meaning of that phrase. Thus, to supply each an equal share of medical goods and services—the most elementary form of distribution—seems unjust and simplistic. Such a formula would treat dissimilar situations in the same fashion, allotting shares equally to the hemophiliac and the vigorous and healthy. Once this simplistic ideal of justice has been abandoned, however, it is unclear what appropriate indices for allocation ought to be employed. To each according to—what? In the following discussion, we will consider the major contenders which bid to perform the role of measuring justice: (1) ability to pay; (2) individual merit; (3) social worth; and (4) need.[6] We will argue for a system which favors need as the measure of just medical care allocation. We will also indicate how need must be seen in the context of the community, and defined by the community, rather than be left to the personal definitions, whims, or idiosyncrasies of patients or physicians.

Market Justice

The dominant notion of justice in American medicine has followed the general American model: to each according to his ability to satisfy wants and needs in the open market of supply and demand. In short, to each according to his ability to pay. Dan Beauchamp has termed this idea "market justice," and noted that it emphasizes individual responsibility, minimal collective action, and freedom from communal obligations. He argues that market justice has undermined our ability to protect the public's health, and that it perpetuates high instances of early death and disability in America.[7]

Those more favorably impressed with market measures of justice have generally argued for it in the tradition of individualism and absolute rights described earlier. Robert Sade, for example, in a well-known article in the *New England Journal of Medicine* in 1972, presented a case for market justice by arguing against a right to health care. Sade's position is that since a physician owns his professional skills, he is entitled to dispense them as he pleases. As bread belongs to the baker who made it, to sell at whatever price he wishes, so medical services belong to the physician. To force the physician into a fee schedule, or to oblige him to see patients he does not choose, is to violate the physician's liberty and his right to practice as he sees fit.[8]

Justice is served when the free market is preserved. If a physician chooses to serve those who cannot pay, it is a charitable act, but not one which is in any sense required by any other authority than the autonomous self who freely chooses to act in this fashion.

Sade represents only the most blatant expression of a system which has long dominated American medicine. The evidence for this judgment is that the major medical care reforms, either contemplated or enacted over the past two decades, have assumed the validity of market justice and sought to extend and amplify its influence over medical access and distribution. Medicare and Medicaid are the most visible examples of public subsidy for private markets to correct for inequities in service. National health insurance plans (as proposed to date) are more of the same genre of remedy. Rather than alternatives to market justice, they are extensions of it since none of the basic assumptions of the free enterprise paradigm are challenged. The sort of tinkering which has been done, in fact, only increases and affirms the hold of market paradigms over the American imagination.

Yet the idea of market justice is deeply flawed. "To each according to ability to pay" does not serve us well in medical care for four basic reasons.

1. The first reason is that persons are hardly in a bargaining position when they are ill or injured. Persons seek a physician when they are compromised—functionally, physically, psychologically. They are emphatically not free, rational agents in the market, able to barter and choose intelligently among the services available to them. As only one example, distance and transportation may severely limit choice for the poor and the aged; indeed, this is a problem even among those of substantial means. Seeking help when one is ill is not like shopping for a shirt or soliciting bids on a building project. The "sick role" entails a somewhat compromised capacity to judge, and it certainly includes restriction on what is optimally only a theoretical range of choices about whom to see and how much to pay for services. The patient as free agent is a questionable metaphor and, we think, largely a fictional account of this reality.

2. The second flaw in the market model of justice is the idea that physicians constitute a supply and demand market. The classic laws of supply and demand do not, in fact, operate in medical care. Indeed, the evidence shows that just the reverse occurs. The greater the supply of physicians, the greater the demands and the greater the cost for medical services. This is so because physicians largely generate

their own business. They are simultaneously the experts who decide
who needs care (gatekeepers) and the recipients of the financial rewards. This dual role provides no incentives for cost control and ex-
acerbates the market difficulties.[9] The sometimes-cited image of the
unemployed physician who drives a cab because of oversupply has
proved fictitious to date.

The point here is that the medical care system enjoys a monopoly,
that physicians are largely bound to each other by noncompetitive,
fraternal ties, and that the financial controls of the system are still
largely in the hands of individual practitioners. The market ideology
does not fit the facts.

3. The third reason that market justice does not serve us well is
that it contains a hidden merit criterion for access to care. "To each
according to ability to pay" functions on the premise that those who
have succeeded in the social order will, indeed, have the money to
pay. Those without money to buy services, it is assumed, have not
succeeded; and it is frequently assumed, largely because of their own
behavior. Market justice rewards those with financial resources and
disenfranchises further those who lack such resources. Market justice
follows, and accepts as normative, the economic disparities that already exist in society. Market justice says that disparities of wealth
translate into disparities of health. It sees this as unfortunate, but not
unfair. As we will discuss later, the cycle of bad health and lack of
money, in which each condition feeds upon and worsens the other, is
ignored by the free market paradigm.

4. The fourth and final flaw in market justice is the most intimate
to the practitioner. It is expressed forcefully by Sade as one of ownership of professional skills. The source of this idea is, again, John
Locke, whose notions of ownership have figured so powerfully in the
American mind. Locke contended that one is entitled to ownership in
anything which is removed from the state of nature by one's own labor. Applied to medicine, this means that by virtue of the labor of
education and practice, the individual physician owns his skills and,
as Sade contends, can dispense with them as he would any private
property.

On reflection, the oddity of this idea becomes apparent. To say, "I
own my professional skills," implies a degree of distance which is
antithetical to our sense of professionalism. To say, "I own my professional skills," can, of course, take on a sense of negative reference;
as if to say, no one else owns them, the government doesn't own

them, and so on. Yet, as a positive statement, the assertion seems like a grammatical misfire. My professional skills are not owned by me; they are me. They are not my property (except in some misanthropic sense); rather, they are part of my self-understanding. It is surely awkward and inappropriate to say, "I have professional skills, which I own, for sale." We are (dare we say!) more naturally inclined to say simply, "I am a professional," or, "I am a doctor." It is this deeper sense of professional authority and skills, held as a public trust and in the service of the public good, that has made the professions what they are. Sade's interpretation, based on a private property model, would vitiate the professions entirely and destroy the sort of prerogatives which he is otherwise so intent on protecting. These prerogatives—to the extent that they are legitimate—are grounded in commitment to service above the desire for personal gain; they are not rooted in questions of ownership.

For these reasons, market justice is a failure. The other measures of justice we will consider more briefly.

Merit Justice

"To each according to success or achievement," if merit is measured in dollars, is just a variation of the market model. But, as one of the major contenders for measuring justice in the distribution of scarce medical resources and services, merit is customarily viewed in terms of the effort to keep healthy. It usually refers, therefore, to individual behaviors which are designed to foster health maintenance.

Those who favor a system of distribution based on merit are concerned with the extent to which disease and illness are brought upon oneself by lifestyle. Cases in which personal habits or choices make persons users of medical resources are well known and range from the correlations between cigarette smoking and lung cancer, or obesity and cardiovascular disease, to the risks associated with hanggliding, motor racing, and mountaineering.

We know that a vast number of disabilities, illnesses, and deaths—due to causes not always beyond our control—do occur each year; and we believe, in view of this evidence, that people do have an effect on—and therefore a responsibility for—their own medical needs. Insofar as lifestyles influence mortality and morbidity, there is substantial appeal in the merit argument for medical care distribution. But to stop here would oversimplify the process of assigning responsibility, as well as inflate our knowledge of causes. Most illnesses are not attributable to either a microbe or a bad habit, a germ or a personal choice of lifestyle; and we now recognize that the causes of illness are multiple, and their lines of influence and interaction very complex.

In recognition of the far-from-simple etiology of illnesses, it *could* be argued that attributing illness to lifestyle and voluntary risk ought to determine allocation in another fashion: more resources should be devoted to prevention and other interventions *before* rather than after the fact!

Whatever we do to alter lifestyles and hazardous choices, and however threatening the illnesses and injuries from these causes may become, there remains a broad range of natural contingencies over which we have neither voluntary choice nor power of precise prediction. There is a tragic dimension associated with the human condition which rightly makes us cautious about supposing that we can always, or perhaps even usually, assign differentiated responsibility for life's misfortunes. That is why it would be absurd, in this society, to argue that a newborn deserved his hemophilia and therefore did not merit access to treatment.

In the final analysis, denying effective medical care to those who have deviated from accepted health behaviors has the same effect as the market model: the victim is blamed in both systems. In addition, a too-often neglected (and tacitly denied) aspect of the blaming phenomenon strikes deeper to the heart of corporate social life: in blaming the victim, the rest of society is exonerated from any responsibility. If, to take but one example, cigarette smoking is an entirely individual choice, then tobacco subsidies, advertising, peer pressures, and all those other factors in the social environment which induce people to smoke can be discounted. Both merit and merit justice, for these reasons, are myopic and anti-communal.

Justice as Social Worth

"To each according to societal contribution" is a notion which, unlike merit justice, embodies some requirement to look at larger public and social arrangements and needs. On these terms, priority in medical care is given on the basis of the common good, community welfare, or the greatest good for the greatest number. On the face of it, this index of justice is superior to others we have considered by virtue of its emphasis on the whole community of persons. The most valuable members of a society, according to this approach, should be cared for first. Under this allocation scheme, persons would not be treated as ends in themselves, but as component means to a socially valued end. The President, for example, should receive the best care available, even if that means diverting resources from others. Yet beyond this simple and somewhat obvious case, judging and choosing between or among people, or classes of people, on the grounds of social worth becomes very like trying to climb a greased pole. Two well-known cases are sufficient to establish the point:

(A) Early in the 1960s when renal dialysis was in its infancy and dialysis units were scare, Seattle's Swedish Hospital established a committee to decide which patients, among the large number in need of renal dialysis, would be granted access to the small number of dialysis machines. After certification of "medical acceptability," the criteria adopted by the selection committee were broadly social and economic in nature. The considerations which were weighed included age, gender, marital status, number of dependents, net worth, educational background, occupation, past performance, and future potential. At one time, the committee received letters of reference in order to assist their evaluation of candidates. The application of such criteria proved exceedingly problematic.[10] Should someone with six children have priority over a composer or artist? Were those who had suitably arranged their financial and personal affairs to be penalized for being provident? The committee's process has been roundly criticized for its evident bias in selection; but the most important point is that no process could have been free of bias. The fact of the matter is that social worth judgments about individuals cannot be securely made, and therefore should not be attempted.

To try to assess—on the basis of maleability, frequency of occurrence, or morbidity—which *diseases* should be treated is a different matter. For example, it is not absurd or hopelessly biased to decide, on the basis of available intervention, that some forms of cancer should not be the purview of curative medicine, but of only palliative care. To decide that resources should go into prevention is not to abandon or discriminate against some cancer patients; it is simply to attempt a rational assessment of effective intervention. To fail to attempt such an assessment would be unjust overall.

(B) A somewhat different case involves judgments, not about individuals, but about classes of individuals. Early in World War II, the American authorities decided to reserve penicillin, then new and in short supply, for military casualties. Paul Freund has described the options faced by American officers in a military hospital in North Africa in 1943.[11] There was enough penicillin to treat either, but not both, of two groups of soldiers: those who had been wounded in combat, or those who had contracted venereal disease while on leave. The decision was made to give priority to those with venereal disease, on the grounds that they could be cured more quickly and thus made ready faster for combat.

The point of major interest about this judgment of social worth is that it is not the worth of the men themselves as persons, but their worth to the larger cause of winning the war, that is judged. One could argue, indeed it was argued, that this latter case (unlike the Swedish Hospital case) rests finally on a compelling need—the need for victory and the instrumental worth of soldiers toward its achievement. That judgments of worth, in the larger social list of needs, would result in treating individuals in a purely instrumental way is, to be sure, not without problems. Therefore, the list of societal needs tends to be fairly clear in time of war or national emergency; otherwise, decisions are rarely so simple. In a time of scarcity and competition for goods and services, the hazard is ever-present that needs can easily conflate into value judgments of the superior worth of certain segments of the population over others.

As we have seen, no matter what criteria of selection are used, it is the inherently prejudicial nature of the selection process which is problematic. Market justice, merit justice, and justice as social worth are each flawed by the overt or covert values which are inextricably bound up in them. The presence of value components is not the problem; the problem is that money, merit, and social worth are the wrong values to employ in resolving this conflict. Instead of achieving justice in medical care, the use of these criteria deforms and cripples justice. These measures, while they may well have a proper sphere of application, do not work appropriately for medical care allocation. Business transactions should not be based on need, nor awards made on the basis of ability to pay, nor medical care distributed on the basis of social worth. Each of these represents the application of a value outside its appropriate sphere of influence. The natural criterion for just distribution of medical care, we think, is need.

Needs, Desires, and Individual Liberties

The criterion of need has been implicit as a second requirement of each of the measures of justice discussed above. What we affirm here is *need alone* as the measure of just distribution of medical care: to each according to his need. Ill health is the sort of thing which is unevenly distributed and over which we can exercise, at best, only moderate control; medical care should therefore be distributed on the basis of need. Ingredient in our recognition of need as the sole desideratum is the fact that access to medical care, when needed, is precursor to almost every other good which society can offer—work, professional advancement, housing, food, opportunities for cultural enrichment, and the like. Illness is not just one burden among others; it is also a condition of injured or compromised human agency. The sick live in the dark side of the human condition, and to deny them access to effective medical care is to write off their existence as persons. Because good medical care can be, and often is, foundational for any real sense of social functioning in our society, it should be distributed on the basis of need alone.

It has been suggested that, far from being a clear indicator, "need" is just as slippery a slope and subject to abuse as "social worth." But this is true only if the notion of need is left to the caprice and whimsy of individual doctors or patients. If "need" be seen as the private and relative possession of individuals, it cannot help but succumb to such abuse. This, however, does not have to happen; and we turn now to an alternative point of view.

Need, we argue, is the only relevant criterion for choosing between individuals, or classes of individuals. This does not imply that all needs can or should be met. Indeed, in times of scarce resources, perhaps only a minimally decent standard of medical needs can be met. Reasonable people would agree that even meeting minimal standards in medical care must be weighed against other social needs, such as food, housing, education, or national defense. So medical care is not society's only need; but for medical care, need alone is the criterion for just distribution. Whatever system of care is available should be equally available without regard for money, merit, or other social worth barriers.

The necessity to delineate carefully the range of genuine needs in this society comes, ironically, at a time in which we seem to be moving in the direction of omnibus medicine. Since the abandonment by Western medicine of the classical warrant for medical intervention (namely, the presence of a definitely diagnosed physiologic lesion which is believed to be pathologic), and the introduction of psychological and psychiatric warrants for intervention, it has become much easier for the omnicompetent model of medical care to function. We do not mean, nor do we want, to say that modern medicine must be limited by the older warrant for intervention; yet prophylactic mastectomy, rhinoplasty, deep electrode implantation for the control of violence, lobotomy, lobectomy, hysterectomy, breast augmentation, hip reduction, and other procedures which are currently fashionable raise questions. Can we any longer discriminate between serious and frivolous medical interventions except on the grossest terms of a social utility?

If there is no longer an agreed-upon way by which the public interest monitors behavior, and if private freedom is understood chiefly as noninterference, the common good can assert itself only by oppressing individual liberty. Without rational canons by which we adjudicate what is needful and desirable from what is not, professional service becomes severely politicized. That divisions run very deep over how these questions will be answered only confirms the urgency and the high stakes signified by asking whether there are any limits or boundaries to competent medical interventions in these areas; and, if so, whether those boundaries will be measured by need justice rather than some other criteria we have discussed.

We have thus far been loath in this country, certainly in formal arguments, to affirm social utilitarianism as either the necessary or the sufficient criterion for health care services. But we also perpetuate a fee-for-service system which discriminates among the recipients of medical care according to the ability to pay.

Simultaneously, many Americans have abdicated a large measure of responsibility for their own health and, accordingly, transferred many of their expectations for the good life to ever-expanding medical intervention. Rescue medicine is the systemic answer to that abdication and transfer. All the same, there is not much doubt among people who have worried over these things that we cannot do everything for everybody, and that we will soon have to face squarely the hard choices regarding scarce or costly resources and personal privilege in terms of limiting demand. Those limitations, as all decisions in this society which set boundaries on individual freedoms, will not be easy either to identify or to impose; and both the ethical warrants and the public policies which venture to address these matters will probably be painful and troublesome to extract.

To this point in our nation's history, we have generally affirmed the libertarian rhetoric that each of us is able, within our own resources and preferences, to set our own private lifestyle with minimal interference from others. Our growing interdependency and the scarcity of services and goods bid fair to change that. How tractable we are toward such change will be a major test of our humanity.

Among the possible ways in which some of these changes might occur, two are worth mentioning here. The first we will call "benevolent paternalism" (with emphasis on benevolent). We may soon decide that society has a larger stake than it has heretofore acknowledged in protecting persons from themselves. The principle which warrants such an encroachment on private freedom is not at issue—we already have compulsory schooling, inoculations, and taxes. What is at issue is how far we will go and into what areas.

To cite a matter which is currently volatile in the policy arena, consider whether it might ever be appropriate to limit the number of elective abortions available to a woman, not because of controversy over payment schemes or the status of fetal life but in recognition of the several contraindicating sequelae which follow from multiple scarrings of the endometrium. There is, in fact, precedent for limiting personal freedom in this way, as attested to by statutes which provide for involuntary commitment and involuntary sterilization.

An alternative, which we will call "forebearing egalitarianism," is to extend the ways in which society is protected from some of its citizens; principally, let us say, through discontinuance or unavailability of some high-technology and costly procedures. To take this step would require us to say, in effect: you are free to engage in a lifestyle which, in our best judgment, is conducive to certain diseases and disorders and injuries; but if you become a victim, you cannot expect to be rescued by public resources.

To make decisions of this sort quietly and covertly is our usual practice; but to suggest them *openly* is to invite ridicule and wrath because they appear altogether inimical to cherished notions of utilitarianism, individualism, autonomy, and noninterference. Those notions have come to us bound together in a system of thought which is commonly attributed to John Stuart Mill. In his famous essays, *Utilitarianism* and *On Liberty,* Mill stated that:

actions are right in proportion as they tend to promote happiness, wrong as they tend to produce the reverse of happiness. By happiness is intended pleasure, and the absence of pain; by unhappiness, pain, and the privation of pleasure.[12]

the sole end for which mankind are warranted, individually or collectively, in interfering with the liberty of action of any of their number, is self-protection . . . the only purpose for which power can be rightfully exercised over any member of a civilized community, against his will, is to prevent harm to others. His own good, either physical or moral, is not a sufficient warrant. . . . In the part which merely concerns himself, his independence is, of right, absolute. Over himself, over his own body and mind, the individual is sovereign.[13]

The thesis of Mill's essays is that the greatest happiness for the greatest number will flow from a policy of absolute nonintervention in the private affairs of individuals, and from a policy of strictly qualified interference in the public affairs of individuals. Thus, society must never interfere in the private affairs of individuals, even for the purpose of making the same individuals happier! That seems nonsensical, because it defeats the purpose of noninterference, which is to achieve the greatest happiness; and one would have thought that one way to increase the sum of happiness would be to interfere in ways both to produce happiness and to prevent unhappiness. But that, according to Mill, is inappropriate because each person is sovereign over the definition of happiness and unhappiness.

What has happened, for both Mill and his libertarian heirs, is that individualism has ceased to be a means and become an end in itself; or, to put it differently, liberty no longer functions instrumentally toward the achievement of happiness or some other goal, but is itself the terminal value. This is individualism for individualism's sake, freedom for freedom's sake; and the suspicion that Mill actually valued individualism for itself, and merely defended it by a utilitarian argument, is thereby convincingly reinforced. In the final analysis, Mill's legacy to American democratic political liberalism is that the individual is the best judge of his own interests, indeed the *only* judge of his own interests.

That would be clear enough, had Mill left the matter there; but the issue gets confused by introduction of the utilitarian calculus and Mill's concession that some individuals who commit certain acts cannot possibly be in full possession of their faculties, and therefore are rightly regarded as children, madmen, or idiots, and rightly treated as wards of the society! These latter qualifications violate in principle the right of the individual to make his own decisions, even at the risk of ruining himself or losing his life, and the doctrine of individual freedom is thereby so much diminished as to make its claim or viability *dependent* upon public beneficence rather than independent as a function of individual rights. Mill himself realized that the doctrine of absolute nonintervention could not be defended on utilitarian grounds; and in the concluding chapter ("Of the Grounds and Limits of the Laissez-faire or Non-Interference Principle") of his essay on the *Principles of Political Economy,* he recognized at least seven sorts of cases in which government intervention can be justified in order to achieve the greatest happiness by serving the general welfare.[14] Thus, although committed to a utilitarianism which was methodologically individualistic, Mill himself acknowledged the inadequacy of the individualistic model for achieving human happiness within social relationships.

The issue—in some sense, the problem—which social justice addresses to American medical care was succinctly stated some years ago by Edgar Friedenberg: "American society is not designed to respond to needs, which is what losers have. Instead, it responds to demands, which are what winners are in a position to make."[15] Justice per se is concerned with needs as the primary datum for worrying about fairness and proportionality and equity; and its prominence in our cultural history is as ancient as the Hebrew prophets or as current as the most recently enacted welfare statute. The subject matter of justice, in other words, are the "losers": that is, the people in this society who are not only economically deprived and disadvantaged but who are also, largely as a function of that anterior reason, deprived and disadvantaged in other aspects of their existence. For our purposes here, those "other aspects" focus preeminently on medical care. We believe that this is an urgent matter of business in this society, if only because it is such a long-neglected item on the national agenda.

Medical Care and the Culture of Poverty

The most obvious evidence of need in this society is poverty, but impecuniousness is only one of the marks of this condition. In fact, a lack of money is also typically one's ticket to poor education, poor employment, poor performance, and poor incentive as well as inferior nutrition, hygiene, and health. So the presumption that economics alone lies at the root of this problem is mistaken. If we simply suppose that money or goods or services, or any combination of these, will provide an adequate solution to the problem of poverty in an affluent and acquisitive society, we will fail to comprehend the many subtle and insidious faces of poverty, the range of injustice and oppression compassed by that condition, and the reasons that poverty is a problem at all. Indeed, poverty constitutes a condition pervasive enough in lifestyle, rituals, myths, and a structure of belief systems to be called a culture.[16]

Being poor—that is, being needy, weak, insufficient, or lacking—is a universal human condition; and that is why each of us, if we compare another's gift or possessions or capabilities with our own, is poor. But what makes economic destitution simultaneously so basic and pervasive is that, in this society, it is increasingly the case that possession of money is precursory to virtually everything else that the society has to offer. Of course we continue to celebrate the Horatio Alger myth as an indispensable element of the American dream; and on occasion somebody seems to have had the serendipitous coincidence of good luck, resourcefulness, ability, and opportunity to make that dream come true. Actually, for the large majority of Americans, the possibility itself has never been much more than a formal potential, and the economic history of the nation tends to confirm that, on the whole, the rich become richer and the poor become poorer.

To be sure, we have made remarkable, gigantic strides in scientific and technical achievement, in gross national product, and in attaining the highest standard of living in human history. Even so, the differential between the poor and the rest of us remains fairly constant. Moreover, the ethical dilemmas of this society are not rooted in that kind of progress; neither do the moral crises that confront us emerge from the risks which attend our scientific accomplishments or the perils which accompany the promise of our technological triumphs.

Our ethical dilemma is, first of all, that we cannot or will not agree upon a common set of values that take poverty seriously; and, second, that we have no firm consensus as to what is true and good and just; and, third, that we cannot any longer (if we ever could) assume that we share common notions of duties and rights. Our moral crises derive from that ethical heteronomy: because we cannot agree upon the principles of virtue, we are in conflict about the practice of virtue.

The problem of poverty, together with the several disabilities which accompany and reinforce it, has arisen and remains unsolved in this society because of an idolatry: in this case, wealth and the power which attends it are valued over persons and their varied human needs. Were it not for our commitment and devotion to existing economic arrangements and professionalized institutions, novel ideas and ways and means of organizing and managing wealth and of eradicating poverty might emerge. But our great difficulty in imagining alternatives only indicates the measure to which the old idols hold us captive. Poverty comes into being because of a distorted perspective on private property, the place of work in society, the use of wealth, and the relative value of persons and machines. That is why poverty is a human problem, amenable to human solutions, and not attributable to any other incapacity or impotence than the sheer human permission to maintain this affliction amid affluence, and the dreadful waste of human promise and potential which follows in its wake.

It would seem reasonable that *financial access* is the villain of this piece; indeed, for most of us the main problem is affording to buy what we need from an ever-lengthening list of high-quality medical care goods and services. But Leonard Schifrin, a medical economist, has shown that financial access, as we have arranged it for the poor, is at best a mixed blessing. While Medicaid and Medicare have surely raised the medical care consumption patterns and utilization levels of the poor, resolution of financial access of the poor

does not end their health care problems, by a wide margin. First, because the poor have substandard health, equalizing their access to health care does not come to grips with their relatively greater needs or to the circumstances that tend to generate their low health conditions. Second, the poor in our society face barriers to good health care other than financial ones, and these barriers have not been reduced or removed to any degree comparable with the lowering of the financial barriers. Perhaps we see here the anomaly of the typical American solution to societal problems: reallocate income or, what is the same thing, spend generously of public funds, but demonstrate a strong reluctance to alter in any significant way the basic institutional conditions that create the problem.[17]

To put this in terms of Slater's parable, the problem is not our resources or our ingenuity, but the absence of social imagination.

Primary Care as Social Justice

Social justice should be a natural initial concern of the primary care physician, not an afterthought or a second order of professional responsibility. It is, of course, true that physicians care for patients one at a time, and that every physician-patient relationship is unique and individualized. Yet the distinction between individual and social ethics is somewhat artificial and exaggerated in America; in whatever sense the two may be distinguished, they cannot finally be separated. Patients do not enter the clinic as isolated diseases or even as discrete psychosocial units. They dwell in a cultural system, with an interpersonal history, in a social hierarchy, and are participant in a larger political environment. None of these can be ignored or dismissed except on pain of denying the patient as person. Our concern is that the social dimension of these personal therapeutic alliances has been underestimated and, hence, undervalued.

There are, in addition, special ways that justice is a concern of the primary care practitioner. As we indicated in chapter 3, the rejection of Aesculapian authority as a paradigm for patient care bespeaks a concern for the accessibility and acceptability of medical services as called for in the Institute of Medicine definition of primary care. This concern is, in itself, an implicit acceptance of social justice as a legitimate item on the professional agenda. Knowledge of the symbiotic relationship between individual access and larger social maladies such as poverty gives these laudatory phrases real meaning. The recognition that poverty is not merely a contingent condition, but a perpetuated, cultural subsystem in America, should make us wary of any effort merely to make minor adjustments in the system. To achieve justice in access requires more thoroughgoing reform of the system itself.

Moreover, it is essential to remember that primary care is a mode of viewing medical services. While respecting the tertiary care picture of rescue medicine, primary care sees medical services as ways of caring for, alleviating, coping with, and containing illness when cure is questionable or impossible. The value, both material and symbolic, of these functions is considerable.

Primary care physicians should have a special stake in just distribution of medical services because of their proximity to the social fabric of illness and because of their commitment to care, even when cure is beyond reach.

Finally, as Pellegrino and Thomasma have indicated, primary care is fundamentally a form of personal security for patients.[18] It implies patient advocacy in a large and complex system of care; it provides, or should provide, constancy in interacting with the system of hospitals and consultants. Primary care is primary in the sense that the patient's welfare is first and foremost, but it is also primary in the sense of entry or first contact with medicine. It is this responsibility for keeping the gate which makes attention to social justice, as well as to personal virtue, so important for both the primary care physician and the public at large.

Our concern with social justice as a part of primary care ethics does not mean that we think doctors should become social reformers and forsake their role as healers. For the physician, social justice is always focused at the point of rendering care to patients, one at a time. The traditional ethics of medicine is so exclusively concerned with individuals, however, that social justice questions tend to become invisible. The passage from one patient's care to the social ethos in which care is rendered must become transparent. This transparency is not at all inimical to good individual care, as it is often portrayed; instead, it puts patient care in proper perspective. Individual and social ethics do not conflict, but are the same obligations with a different focus. Depending upon the focus, the ill person can be a specimen of pathological tissue, or a victim of poverty or some other social pathology.

It is not our aim here to speculate about the actions which practitioners individually or collectively should undertake to achieve a larger measure of justice. We do not believe that major changes will be possible until the social dimensions of illness are better appreciated; and we know that there are major conceptual barriers which block such appreciation. We have tried to indicate what some of these barriers are, and also to indicate how deeply they lie within the American sensibility. We have also tried to show that, by its own definition, primary care medicine is an instrument of social justice. How effective it will be is a question to be addressed at some future date.

For the present we wish to reaffirm the moral vision which lies at the core of primary care medicine. The specific responsibilities of primary care practitioners will become more clear as we attempt to respond to the prior question of justice: To what sort of moral community do physicians and patients belong?

Notes

Introduction

1. This case, together with others, will be discussed in chapter 4.

2. Tom Beauchamp and James Childress, *Principles of Biomedical Ethics,* 2d ed. (New York: Oxford University Press, 1983).

1. Primary Care: A Moral Notion

1. Wendy Carlton, *In Our Professional Opinion . . . The Primacy of Clinical Judgment over Moral Choice* (South Bend: University of Notre Dame Press, 1978).

2. This case, together with others, will be discussed in chapter 4.

3. Eric D'Arcy, *Human Acts: An Essay on Their Moral Evaluation* (New York: Oxford University Press, 1963), p. 18.

4. We must return to examine the adequacy and accuracy of these modifiers in this context. Whether these and other technologies are indeed "life supportive" or "death deferring" may make significant ethical difference when such an action as withdrawal or stoppage is undertaken.

5. Paul Ramsey, *Deeds and Rules in Christian Ethics* (New York: Scribners, 1967), pp. 197–198.

6. J. J. Alpert and E. Charney, "The Education of Physicians for Primary Care," U.S. DHEW, Publication No. (HRA) 74-3113 (1973).

7. A. Janeway, "The Decline of Primary Medical Care: An Unforeseen Consequence of the Flexner Report," *Pharos* (July 1974): 74–80.

8. H. K. Silver, and P. R. McAtee, "A Descriptive Definition of the Scope and Context of Primary Health Care," *Pediatrics* 56 (1975): 957.

9. R. G. Petersdorf, "Issues in Primary Care: The Academic Perspective," *Journal of Medical Education* 50 (December 1975): 5–13.

10. John S. Millis, "Primary Care: Definition of, and Access to . . . ," *Nursing Outlook* 25 (July 1977): 443–445.

11. David E. Rogers, "The Challenge of Primary Care," *Daedalus* 106 (Winter 1977): 81–103.

12. David E. Rogers, "Primary Care: Some Issues," *Bulletin of the New York Academy of Medicine* 53 (January/February 1977): 10–17.

13. Ibid.

14. J. F. Mustard, Chairman, "Report of the Health Planning Task Force," Ontario Ministry of Health (Toronto, January 28, 1974), p. 27.

15. American Academy of Family Physicians, Official Document No. 302. January 30, 1976.

16. "A Glossary for Primary Care," Report of the North American Primary Care Research Group (NAPCRG) Committee on Standard Terminology, *Journal of Family Practice* 5 (October 1977): 633–638. This definition is clearly indebted to the AAFP's definition, as similarly the NAPCRG's definition of "health" ("The state of optimal physical, mental, and social well-being and not merely the absence of disease or infirmity") is a revised version of the World Health Organization's definition.

17. E. Harvey Estes (Chairman) et al., "A Manpower Policy for Primary Health Care," Institute of Medicine, National Academy of Sciences (1978), IOM Publication 78-02, p. 1.

2. Ethics and Professionalism

1. Of course, Bacon is not the only one responsible for this revolution, but he may well be the example *par excellence* in the same way that, were we talking about cognition and epistemology rather than scientific method, we could focus attention on René Descartes.

2. Paul Ramsey, *The Patient as Person* (New Haven: Yale University Press, 1970), p. 1.

3. Louis Lasagna, "Some Ethical Problems in Clinical Investigation," in *Human Aspects of Biomedical Innovation,* ed. Everett Mendelsohn, Judith Swazey, and Irene Toviss (Cambridge: Harvard University Press, 1971), p. 108.

4. Edmund Pellegrino, "Physicians, Patients and Society: Some New Tensions in Medical Ethics," ibid., p. 94.

5. Robert Merton, George Reader, and Patricia Kendall, eds., *The Student Physician: Introductory Studies in the Sociology of Medicine* (Cambridge, Mass.: Harvard University Press, 1957).

6. The Declaration of Independence and Amendments 5 and 14 to the Constitution.

7. Arthur Dyck, "Ethics and Medicine," *The Linacre Quarterly* 40 (August 1973): 182–200.

8. Robert Veatch, "Medical Ethics: Professional or Universal?" *Harvard Theological Review* 65 (October 1972): 531–559.

9. Clifford Geertz, *The Interpretation of Cultures* (New York: Basic Books, 1973), p. 127.

10. Miriam Siegler and Humphrey Osmond, "Aesculapian Authority," *Hastings Center Studies* 1 (1973): 41–52.

11. Talcott Parsons, *The Social System* (New York: The Free Press of Glencoe, 1951), pp. 428–447.

12. Edmund Pellegrino, *Humanism and the Physician* (Knoxville: University of Tennessee Press, 1979), p. 119.

13. John McKnight, "Professionalized Service and Disabling Help," in *Disabling Professions,* Ivan Illich, John McKnight, et al. (Salem, N.H.: Marion Boyers, 1977), pp. 69–91.

14. McKnight elaborates the potent political symbolism of talking in these terms by calling attention to several programs which have embraced this language, e.g., *Medi*care, *Edu*care, and *Judi*care. Confirmation is as close as the daily newspaper; ours recently cited with approbation an agency which is engaged in occupational medicine and providing a "new program of professional care" for tenants in a nearby industrial research park. The name? Occucare!

15. Ibid., pp. 4–5.

16. Ibid., p. 19.

17. *Opinions and Reports of the Judicial Council,* American Medical Association (1971), p. 53.

3. Moral Imagination and Medicine

1. Michael Novak, "The Liberation of Imagination," *Man and Medicine* 1 (1976): 107.

2. Luke 10:30–35.

3. Judith Jarvis Thomson, "A Defense of Abortion," *Philosophy and Public Affairs* 1 (1971): 47–66.

4. Raymond Duff, "Guidelines for Deciding Care of Critically Ill or Dying Patients," *Pediatrics* 64 (1979): 17.

5. The Greek word in Luke, which we translate "compassion," is ἐσπλαγχνίσθη and means to have pity, or feel sympathy. The *Oxford English Dictionary* defines "compassion" as "suffering together with another; participating in suffering; fellow-feeling." In this connection, it is interesting that "patient" derives from the Latin *pati,* which means to suffer.

6. Estes et al., "A Manpower Policy for Primary Health Care," pp. 16ff.

7. Michael Foucault, *The Birth of the Clinic,* trans. A. Sheridan Smith (New York: Random House, 1973), p. 97.

8. A. Kleinman, L. Eisenberg, and B. Good, "Culture, Illness and Care: Clinical Lessons from Anthropological and Cross-Cultural Research," *Annals of Internal Medicine* 88 (1978): 251–258.

9. "Three-year Trend of Rx Dept Activity" (Annual Survey), *American Druggist* (May 1980): 18.

10. Leon Kass, "Ethical Dilemmas in the Care of the Ill," *Journal of the American Medical Association* 244 (1980): 1816.

11. *Hippocratic Corpus,* Decorum, XVI: "Perform all this calmly and adroitly, *concealing most things from the patient* while you are *attending to him.* Give necessary orders with cheerfulness and serenity, *turning his attention away* from what is being *done to him;* sometimes reprove sharply and emphatically, and sometimes comfort with solicitude and attention, *revealing nothing of the patient's future or present condition.* For many patients through this cause have taken a turn for the worse, I mean by the declaration I have mentioned of what is present, or by a forecast of what is to come." (Italics added.)

12. Cf. "The Nuremberg Code," in *Trials of War Criminals before the Nuremberg Military Tribunals under Control Council Law No. 10,* vol. 2 (Washington: U.S. Government Printing Office, 1949), pp. 181–182.

13. Pellegrino, *Humanism and the Physician,* p. 227.

14. Iris Murdoch, *The Sovereignty of Good* (London: Routledge and Kegan Paul, 1970), pp. 1–45.

15. Ramsey, *Patient as Person.*

4. Case Studies in Primary Care

1. A. de Saint-Exupéry, *Pilote de guerre* (New York: Editions de la Maison française, 1942), p. 174.

2. William F. May, *The Physician's Covenant* (Philadelphia: Westminster Press, 1983). We may well be extending the use of May's images in ways he would not approve in our analysis, but the use we make of them is suggested by his book.

3. Alasdair MacIntyre, *After Virtue* (South Bend: University of Notre Dame Press, 1981), p. 6ff.

4. For a thorough discussion of the definition and ethics of placebos, see Howard Brody's *Placebos and the Philosophy of Medicine* (Chicago: University of Chicago Press, 1977).

5. Michael Balint, *The Doctor, His Patient and the Illness* (New York: International Universities Press, 1957), pp. 215–238.

5. Primary Care and Social Justice

1. Philip Slater, *The Pursuit of Loneliness,* rev. ed. (Boston: Beacon Press, 1976), pp. xiii–xiv.

2. John Locke, *Two Treatises of Government,* ed. with introduction and notes by Peter Laslett (Cambridge: Cambridge University Press, 1967). See especially Locke's "Second Treatise," and cf. the rhetoric (chiefly Thomas

Jefferson's) in the Declaration of Independence and the Bill of Rights. Locke himself never employed the phrase, "natural rights," nor did he argue any analogy between the laws of nature and the laws of the state; when he argued for natural or fundamental rights, he appealed instead to what is intuitively self-evident, namely that every man has a property in his own person to which nobody but himself has any right. Thus, in Locke's view, the "state of nature" is a condition in which atomic individuals experience natural liberty to be left free to do as one pleases.

3. Ronald Dworkin, *Taking Rights Seriously* (Cambridge, Mass.: Harvard University Press, 1977), p. xi.

4. Stanley I. Benn, "Rights," in *Encyclopedia of Philosophy*, vol. 7 (New York: Macmillan and Free Press, 1967), p. 197.

5. Joel Feinberg, *Social Philosophy* (Englewood Cliffs, N.J.: Prentice-Hall, 1973), pp. 58–67.

6. Our presentation of these measures of justice has been influenced by the perceptive discussion of Gene Outka, "Social Justice and Equal Access to Health Care," in *Journal of Religious Ethics* (Spring 1974): 11–32.

7. Dan E. Beauchamp, "Public Health as Social Justice," *Inquiry* 13, no. 1 (March 1976): 4–6.

8. Robert Sade, "Medical Care as a Right: A Refutation," *New England Journal of Medicine* 286 (1972): 488–493.

9. Alain Enthoven, *Health Plan* (Menlo Park: Addison-Wesley, 1980), pp. 12–30.

10. Cf. Renee C. Fox and Judith P. Swazey, *The Courage to Fail* (Chicago: University of Chicago Press, 1974), esp. chap. 9.

11. Paul Freund, "Organ Transplants: Ethical and Legal Problems," *Proceedings of the American Philosophical Society* 115 (1971): 280.

12. John Stuart Mill, *Utilitarianism, Liberty, and Representative Government* (London: J. M. Dent & Sons, 1910), p. 6.

13. John Stuart Mill, *On Liberty* (London: John W. Parker and Son, 1859), pp. 23–24.

14. John Stuart Mill, *Principles of Political Economy* (London: J. W. Parker, 1848), chap. 11.

15. Edgar Friedenberg, "Bad Blood," in *Readings on Ethical and Social Issues in Biomedicine,* ed. Richard W. Wertz (Englewood Cliffs, N.J.: Prentice-Hall, 1973), pp. 260–268.

16. Oscar Lewis, *La Vida* (New York: Random House, 1966), pp. xlii–lii.

17. Leonard G. Schifrin, "Poverty and Health Care: An Economic Perspective," in *Social Issues in Health Care,* ed. Donnie J. Self (Norfolk: Teagle and Little, 1977), p. 13.

18. Edmund D. Pellegrino and David C. Thomasma, *A Philosophical Basis of Medical Practice* (New York: Oxford University Press, 1981), pp. 242–243.

Index

Library of Congress Cataloging-in-Publication Data
Smith, Harmon L.
Professional ethics and primary care medicine.
Includes index.
1. Medical ethics.   2. Physicians (General practice)
-Professional ethics.   I. Churchill, Larry R.,
45-   . II. Title.   [DNLM: 1. Ethics, Medical.
Primary Health Care—standards.   W 50 S649p]
4.S565   1986   174'.2   85-16098
N 0-8223-0521-6
0-8223-0540-2 (pbk.)